Spunky
Sarah Strydom

Introduction

Publisher's Note

This true story is a snap shot of a difficult time in the life of a little girl - Sarah, or rather Spunky as she is known by her family and friends. Never has a name fitted a person so well.

Sarah at eight years old wrote this book but she was helped by her mother, Nicky. Nicky gave understanding to the medical terms and did the initial edit, but they are Sarah's words.

We have been lenient with the edit for Spunky's words, where we retained incorrect tenses and grammar to preserve her 'voice'.

As the publisher, many have asked me what I enjoyed the most about the manuscript. Obviously Sarah's bravery inspired me, as did her positive outlook. But the best was to get to know Sarah through her candid descriptions. I am sure you will be as enchanted as I was.

I am humbled by the privilege of bringing her story to the world.

Spunky

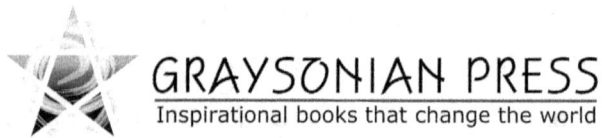

GRAYSONIAN PRESS
Inspirational books that change the world

Published by Graysonian Press

South Africa +27 11 4311274 (0836101113)

Australia 0450260348

www.graysonian.com

pat@graysonian.com

Copyright © Nicky/Sarah Strydom 2012

All rights reserved under international copyright conventions. No part of this book may be reproduced, stored in a retrieval system, or transmitted in any form or by any means electronic, mechanical, photocopying, recorded or otherwise without written permission from Graysonian Press.

Whilst every care has been taken to check the accuracy of the information in this book, the publisher cannot be held responsible for any errors, omissions or originality.

Layout and Cover Design by Ian Stokol

ISBN 978-0-9872816-2-3

Spunky

I want to dedicate this book to my sister Michelle

Testimonial

I clearly remember the first time that I met Sarah. She has that sort of impact on people around her. One just cannot forget her aura, her quiet self-confidence and always the trace of a smile hovering on her face, no matter whether she felt well or ill. It was in July of 2004, and I had just returned to Johannesburg from Shanghai, China the previous day, where I had been overseeing the filming of the 2005 edition of the *Moments in Time* project.

I entered the building of AstraZeneca where the filming was taking place, and moved quietly into the film studio to watch the morning photo-shoot, and to do the video interview of the patient. I heard that the morning's subject was a young girl of eight years old, who was having chemotherapy and treatment for a rare Cancer of her leg called Ewing's Sarcoma, a condition that usually resulted in the amputation of the patient's leg. Sarah still had both of her legs, I was told.

What I saw jolted me out of my fatigue from the trip. In front of me, on the platform used for the shoot, was a beautiful, composed and self-assured young girl, surrounded by the Creative Team. The make-up artist Ronel, putting the finishing touches to her hair and powdering her arms, the stylist Ryno, adjusting her wig, the camera assistant taking the light reading, and the photographer, Jeanne-Claire Bischoff preparing for her composition. There was a buzz in the room, with Sarah the centrepiece of it all, like a seasoned model. Dressed in flowing silk and overlaid pink fabric, hands confidently on her hips, head tilted to her right side, she was the epitome of an experienced and consummate fashion model.

I watched with fascination. Was this the young girl who was fighting the biggest battle of her young life? Or was this someone else?

When the shoot was over, and Sarah took her wig and makeup off for the interview, I saw Sarah's incredible strength, her steadfastness, maturity, the ravages of her fight against this disease, her sense of humour, her spirituality. I saw her bald head, the usual result of the chemotherapy she was having. I saw her limping, one leg being shorter than the other. I saw her humility shine through her quiet determination.

I saw an exceptional human being.

As I spoke to her, all captured by film for the Video documentary that was being shot for that year's launch, it was clear that she was in a class of her own. When asked what her ambitions were for her future, she quietly and without any hesitation answered, " I want to be a singer, an actor and a model". She was sure where she was headed, no matter what life threw at her.

I always wrote the poetry for every patient we filmed for the project, and for Sarah, the words came easily to me, and are below her picture on the Calendar for April 2005:

Testimonials

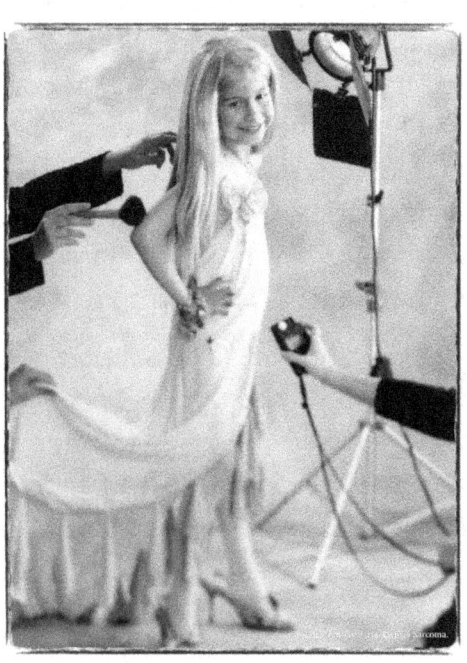

Moments in Time Calendar 2005

*"I know where I'm going, this won't put me back.
Perhaps, in a strange way, it's kept me on track!
Just see what attention life's showering on me
So I can help others be the best they can be".*

Over the many years since then, Sarah has done exactly that... helping others to be the best they can be. Through thick and thin, she has never lost that quiet determination to win through every hurdle. Through surgery, through more treatment, through pain and hardship, she has excelled at sport, she has shown leadership in her social and school circles, she has shown compassion and kindness to many others suffering from one or other form of cancer. On many occasions, when I have spoken about the project *Moments in Time*, to both small and very large audiences, I have asked her to be at my side as an example of what the project stands for, and to speak together with me about her personal journey. Her impact has always been astounding.

With the amazing and dedicated support of her parents, Sarah's life has become a sparkling beacon and a shining light to all who have had the privilege to come into contact with her. She will no doubt continue to lead a very unique and special life as she moves into adulthood. Like very few others, she has epitomised the words of Viktor Frankl, who said that:

"Everything can be taken from a man, except one thing… the last of human freedoms. And that is to choose one's attitude in any given set of circumstances. It is this freedom, which cannot be taken away, that makes life both meaningful and purposeful".

Sarah chose her attitude at a very young age, and she continues to live her dream. She has been a great example to me personally when I have needed strength and repeated validation of how people can and do overcome personal and emotional crises. We write regularly to each other, and she has allowed me to become part of her life. She has fought and won each battle that she has been asked to fight. And she has been steadfast and humble alongside her strength.

Testimonials

I am honoured and privileged to have met her. And I am even more grateful that I can call her my friend.

Professor Matthias Haus

Founder, Director and Past Chairman:
Moments in Time Charitable Trust

May, 2012

The Lump

I was a normal, healthy kid who loved riding my bike and running around. I was clever and enjoyed school. I imagined my life would carry on like this, with nothing going wrong. But everything was going to change.

On Friday the 24 October 2003, Mommy was helping me wash my hair in the bath. I had long blonde hair and hated washing it. I could never get all the shampoo out and combing conditioner through my hair was definitely not my idea of fun. The comb would always get stuck in the knots and often I wished it was shorter just so that I would not battle so much. While Mommy was busy combing my hair she saw a lump on the top of my left leg. It looked a little bit red and slightly swollen.

She asked me, "What happened to your leg? Did you bump yourself or did somebody hurt you?"

It was not sore and I had not noticed it before. I could not remember any bumps or falls that had happened that day. I told her I had not seen it before. We ignored it and rinsed out the conditioner and we carried on chatting about my friends at school. Mommy had to finish cooking dinner and left me to finish washing myself and put on my pyjamas. It was getting warmer and I did not need my dressing gown, my Barbie pyjamas were warm enough. I was hungry and

Spunky

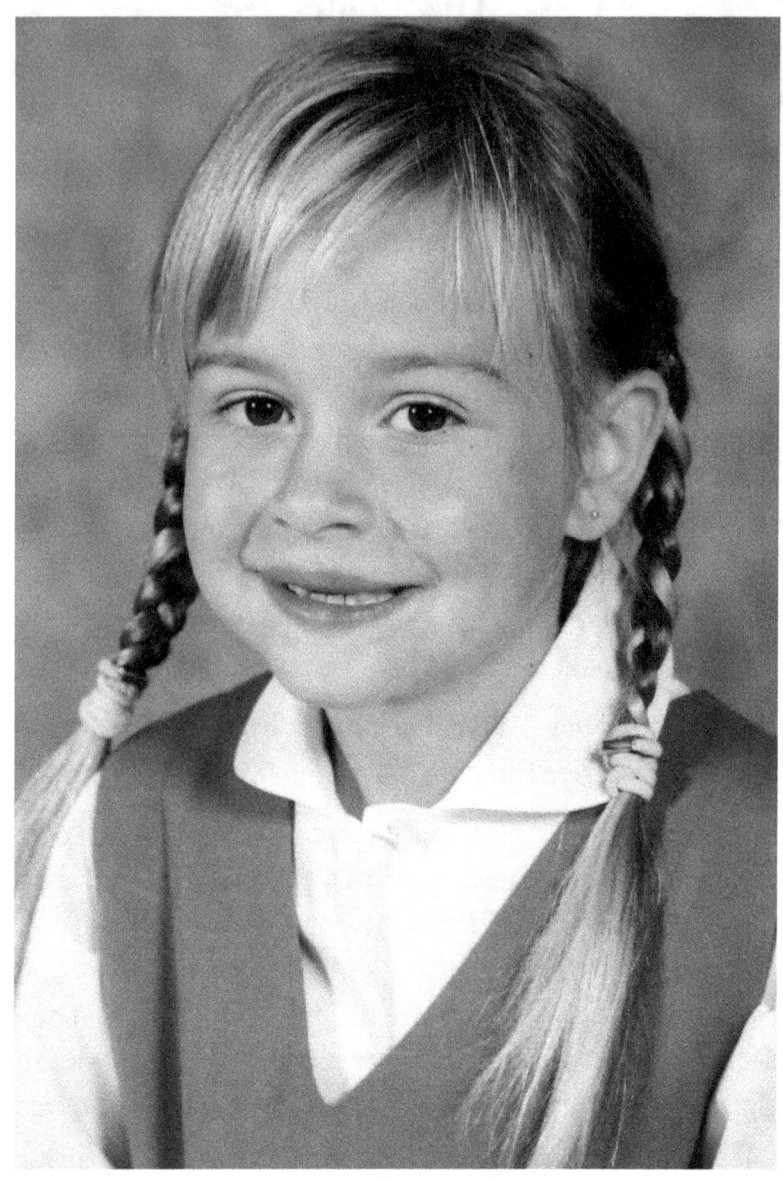

Me at 7 years old

was looking forward to a big plate of macaroni cheese and watching TV. This weekend would be an exciting one, only two more sleeps and it would be my eighth birthday. I was looking forward to my party on Sunday.

The next day while I was getting dressed, Mommy looked at my leg, the strange bump had grown bigger, and you could see many blood vessels. It looked a little bit creepy.

Again she asked me if I had hurt myself and if it was sore. I thought carefully and really couldn't remember anybody hurting me or bumping into anything. I was quite a tomboy and often had bruises and cuts on my legs. That night I could hardly sleep, I was wondering what presents my friends would give me and if everybody I had invited would come to my party.

Finally Sunday arrived, my eighth birthday. I had been looking forward to this day for ages and had that giddy feeling in my tummy from excitement. I woke up really early and I ran into Mommy's bedroom but she and Daddy were still sleeping. I decided to wake up my sister Michelle. We went into the kitchen and made everybody coffee. We took the coffee mugs through to their bedroom, opened the curtains and sat on their bed. Mommy and Michelle went to their cupboards while I sat next to Daddy. They came back with presents for me! We all sat on the bed, it was quite crowded because our three dogs and two cats were also on the bed. I started opening my presents, ripping open the wrapping. Mommy had bought me a new pair of jeans, some brightly coloured T-shirts and some new shoes. I was growing quickly and most of my clothes did not fit anymore. Michelle gave me a beautiful paint-by-number picture. I loved painting! She also gave me the Barbie doll that I had been wanting for ages. I loved Barbie, and loved anything that even had her face on it. I read all the birthday cards and kissed and hugged everybody to thank them. Then Daddy said that there was one more present for me. He asked me to guess where it was. If I got it right, I could have it. I had not been allowed in the garage the whole week and was sure something big was hiding in there. I giggled and guessed the garage. He smiled and told me to go and look. I ran into the garage, switched on the light and there it was. A beautiful shiny blue bicycle. I loved cycling in the streets, it was safe enough then, and I loved ramping the sidewalks and speeding down our road. Daddy opened the garage door and I climbed on my new bike. It was the perfect size, my other bike was too small. I zoomed around the garden at full speed, pretending to be a motorbike racer. I made small tracks in the grass around the house and sped around for ages.

The Lump

Then Mommy called me inside and said I must get ready for the party. I had been so busy riding my bike, I had forgotten about the time and was getting hungry. We ate breakfast and after that we packed the car with all the things we needed for my party. I had invited all my friends to a Zoo Farm, which was close to our house, everybody had replied to say they were coming. I was popular and loved having parties. We patted our dogs and cats goodbye and drove to the zoo farm.

While waiting for everyone to arrive, we walked around looking at some of the animals in the Zoo. Very soon all my friends had arrived, they must have been just as excited as I was.

There was a lot to do there. We rode on ponies and played with the bunnies, fed the horses and wandered around the birdcages, imitating them. There were many animals and we walked around for ages looking at them. I received lots of presents, I was Barbie mad and got a lot of new Barbies and clothes from my friends. I was looking forward to playing with them all. It was so much fun! My whole family was there, all my aunts, uncles and cousins. My cousin gave me a pretty swimming costume, it was red and blue with butterflies on it. Mommy told me to try it on to see that it fitted properly, and I ran to the bathrooms nearby. I was in a hurry because it was very hot and all my friends were waiting for me. They had already changed into their costumes because we were going to run and jump through the sprinklers to cool down. I grabbed my best friend Roxy's hand, eager to try it on, and we both sprinted to the changing rooms.

When I came out of the change rooms, Mommy immediately noticed the lump on my leg. It was the size of a tennis ball. I could not believe how big it had grown. Even my aunt noticed it and asked me what it was. I was not really bothered about it. My new costume fitted perfectly and I ran to join my friends.

A little later Mommy called us, the food was ready.

Hotdogs! My favourite, yummy! We all sat around the big wooden tables, some of my friends were sitting on blankets under the trees. After we had eaten we wandered around the zoo farm again. They had white lions in the cages at the top of the farm. I loved lions and really wanted to see them. We all walked there and when we got back Mommy had put my birthday cake in the middle of the table. Everybody gathered around the table and Mommy lit the candles. I blew them out and then everybody sang "Happy Birthday" to me. Everybody was given a piece of cake and we sat under the trees and ate until our tummies were full.

The Lump

I did not want my party to end. Everybody had a lot of fun and at the end of the day I was sad to say goodbye to my friends. I wanted every day to be like that day.

That night I was very tired and went to bed early. Mommy came to kiss me goodnight. She was still worried about the lump on my leg and how big it had suddenly grown. She told me that she would take me to see Dr Nick the next day. I was not worried, I liked him. He laughed and joked and always gave me a sucker.

"But Mommy, I can't go tomorrow," I suddenly remembered. "Our class is going to the play park tomorrow." The previous week we had a competition at school to see who could raise the most money, I was so excited when my class won. We were going to be rewarded by going to a play park nearby.

"What time are you going there?"

"I don't know and I really don't want to miss it. Please can't we go to Dr Nick some other time? Please Mommy!" I begged.

"Well let's see how your lump is in the morning. If it's smaller, you can go to school." She said as she kissed me goodnight and switched off the light.

The next morning, the lump was still there. I begged Mommy again, she agreed to let me go to the play park for a short time then she would come and fetch me and take me to Dr Nick. This lump really had her worried. I was very excited about going to the play park and quickly got ready for school.

When we got to school, the school bus was waiting for us. My teacher called us all and we lined up to get into the bus. We were allowed to wear civvies (civilian clothes) and on the way to the play park, we sang songs. The morning went by quickly and I was having a lot of fun with my friends when Mommy came to fetch me.

On the way to the doctor's rooms I chatted to Mommy about my fun morning. While we waited to see Dr Nick, Mommy and I paged through a magazine. Soon we were called into his room. Mommy told him about the lump and he had a look at it. He spoke to me and told me that I needed to go to the hospital for a thing he called a 'Sonar Scan'. He wrote out a letter, which Mommy had to take to the hospital. He told Mommy to come back to see him straight after the scan.

On the way to the hospital, Mommy and I chatted about all the presents I got the day before and how much fun my birthday party was. When we got to the hospital, Mommy reminded me that this was the hospital I was born in.

The Lump

A nurse came and called us into the scanning room. Mommy gave her the letter from Dr Nick. The nurse put cold jelly on my leg and used an even colder machine to scan my lump. I could see the picture on the computer screen next to us. The doctor in charge looked very worried and did not say anything to Mommy. He called in four other doctors who crowded around the screen and pointed at something, quietly discussing what they saw. They still did not say anything at all and walked out of the room. The first doctor stayed behind and spoke quietly to Mommy. He told her that the lump was not normal, but suggested that we go for more tests to confirm what it was.

Mommy looked scared and asked him what he thought it was. He said he wasn't sure but said it might be cancerous. He said we must take the results back to Dr Nick. I remember seeing Mommy go white, with big tears in her eyes. The doctor told Mommy to sit down because she was feeling dizzy and was going to faint.

I did not understand why they were looking so sad and kept bugging Mommy to tell me. She told me that she would explain to me when we got into the car. When we walked out of the scanning room, the receptionist asked Mommy if she was going to be okay. Mommy just nodded, with tears streaming down her face.

As soon as we got in the car, I asked Mommy what was going on. She was crying so much she could hardly talk and told me that the doctor thought I might have cancer. I didn't know what that was and asked her. She said it was a very, very serious disease. I also started to cry a bit, but told her that I would be okay and that she mustn't cry so much. I hated seeing Mommy cry, she never cried unless it was really bad.

On the way back to the Dr Nick's rooms, Mommy phoned Daddy and told him what had happened and that he must meet us there. When we arrived, Daddy was already there, also looking very worried. I had never seen Daddy scared before, in my eyes he was always so brave with everything. It was getting late and we were the last patients to see him. He called us into his consulting room and asked for the scan results. He read them carefully. I had never seen him look so sad. Dr Nick was always very happy.

This must be serious but I still did not understand what they were talking about. He told my mom and dad to take me to the Johannesburg General Hospital, the place where my sister, Michelle was born. He said that they had to do more tests and told Mommy to let him know what the results were.

Mom asked him what he thought it was and he also

The Lump

said a cancerous tumour, which made both Mommy and Daddy cry a lot. He gave my mom a letter to take to the Joburg Gen. When we got home, nobody said much. Michelle wanted to know what had happened. After Mommy and Daddy had told her, she also looked worried. I tried to cheer everybody up and told them about the play park. I was looking forward to going back to school and finding out what my friends had done after I had left, but I was worried, seeing everyone was so quiet.

The next day I missed school again. I had to go to the Joburg Gen with Mommy. I had never been in that hospital. It was huge and we got lost.

Eventually we found the Children's Department, where there were hundreds of kids all waiting to see a doctor. Mommy went to a nurse, showed her the letter and asked her if we were in the right place. The nurse told her that we had to go to the Oncology Ward on the ninth floor.

While we walked towards the lifts, I asked Mommy what 'Oncology Ward' meant and she told me it was the cancer ward. I still was not sure what cancer was.

As we got out the lift, Mommy got a phone call from Dr Nick. He wanted to know if we were at the hospital and if we were okay. Mommy told him that we were on our way to the cancer ward. He told her to phone him and let him know what was going to happen. The hospital was so confusing and my mom asked another nurse how to get to the ninth floor because we were lost again.

As we walked into the ward, there were two big creatures in the corner of the room, a big blue Sulley and little Mike from the movie **Monsters Inc**. The ward was full of toys and kids riding little scooters, building puzzles and reading books. It looked so different from the rest of the hospital, which was quite boring. We went to the reception desk and a nurse greeted us with a friendly smile. She introduced herself to us and spoke with a funny accent. She said her name was Sister Susan. She read the letter that Mommy gave her. Then she took us down the corridor and showed us the waiting room. There were many pictures on the walls and toys everywhere. A friendly lady came over and started chatting to me. She asked me my name and how old I was. Then she asked me if I wanted to build a puzzle. I loved puzzles and walked with her to a toy room. There were hundreds of puzzles, books, games and dolls. I chose a puzzle and sat down near Mommy. She chatted to Mommy and explained that she worked for CHOC (Children's Haematology and Oncology Clinic) which was a group of people that would help me and my family get through my treatment.

The Lump

After a while the doctor came and took us through to her consulting room. She was very friendly and joked with me. She asked Mommy what had happened. She read the letter from Dr Nick and then asked me to climb onto the bed. She checked my leg. The lump had grown a bit more and it still looked creepy. I was getting worried because it did not look like it was going away. She pushed on the lump, her hands were a bit cold. She told Mommy that they were going to do a test called a biopsy to see what the lump was. I was not listening to what they were saying and looked around the room. There were lots of pictures on the walls that other kids had painted. There were teddy bears and toys in her room as well.

The doctor was busy telling Mommy that I was in the best possible place to be treated and that she would phone Dr Nick. She told Mommy that I had to come back in three days' time for the biopsy to be done.

I asked her how they did the biopsy, and she explained that they needed to cut out a small piece of my lump and test it, and then they would know what was wrong with me and how to treat it properly. She also explained that I would be off school for a while. Then we went back to the reception desk and made an appointment for three days' time.

It all went dark...

Sister Susan was there and she told Mommy that I would be having an anaesthetic and that I must not eat or drink anything from 10p.m. the night before. She was very friendly and I liked her a lot.

As we walked out of the ward, a kid walked in front of us pushing a drip. She had no hair and looked very sick. I wondered why she was bald. I had a lot of questions for Mommy. I looked at her but she was crying again so I decided to ask her later.

On Wednesday I went back to school to tell my teacher what was happening to me. Mommy went to the staff room to find her but she was not there. She was in the Photostat room and Mommy told her what had happened. I went outside to find my friends. I didn't know that this would be the last time I would see them for a very long time.

Mommy was busy talking to my class teacher and they were both crying. I walked back in and my teacher gave me a big hug. She was pregnant and I did not want to hug her tummy too hard. She could not talk and was choked by tears. Two other teachers walked down the passage and asked what had happened. Mommy told them about my lump and they also started crying.

I really could not understand why everyone was so sad.

That Friday I had to go back to the hospital for my biopsy. I wasn't allowed to eat or drink anything that morning. It was hard because I really wanted a bowl of Pronutro (breakfast cereal) and was starving.

Mommy and Daddy took me back to the ward on the ninth floor. Again we were met by the friendly nurse Sr Susan. She was happy to see us and explained the procedure to my parents. She took me to a ward where there were four other kids, all with their moms or dads.

The one kid in the bed opposite me did not have any hair and looked really pale. Her mom came and spoke to Mommy and told her that it was hectic in the beginning but that all the parents supported each other. She also told Mommy that her daughter had looked the same as me with long blonde hair and was the same age. Mommy could not even talk and was crying again. Then the doctor came in. She was very friendly and explained that I had to go into a small theatre. Only Mommy was allowed to go in with me; Daddy had to wait outside. The nurse gave me a toy crocodile to play with.

Mommy sat next to me on the operating table and held my hand tightly.

"Mommy, I'm scared. Mommy please tell them not to

hurt me, I don't want them to touch me. What are they going to do to me?"

Mommy had explained everything at home but I wanted to find out again.

"They are going to give you an injection so that you go to sleep and don't feel any pain and then they are going to cut out a small piece of the lump and test it. That way they will know what kind of cancer you have and how they are going to treat it. Sarah, you will be fine. Don't worry, I love you and will be here with you through it all. Daddy and I will be waiting for you when you come out of the operation."

An operation? I had never had an operation. Then the nurse put a mask over my mouth and nose and gave me a singing doll to watch while I lay on Mommy's lap. While I listened to the doll sing, tears ran down my face, I was so scared. The nurse asked me to breathe deeply and count. I counted to ten and felt fainter and fainter. Everything became quieter every time I took a breath. I had a funny taste in my mouth, I looked at Mommy, and then… everything went dark.

Mommy had to go outside while they cut a small piece of the tumour out of my leg. Daddy and Sr Susan met her as she walked out of the small theatre. They went into the doctors' tearoom where Sr Susan chatted to Mommy, asking her where she works and about the family. Mommy was not very chatty because she was worried about me. Then she offered my parents some tea and sandwiches.

She explained to them that her daughter had been diagnosed with a very serious blood disease many years ago and that she was now an adult and completely cured. She said that most of the childhood cancers could be treated successfully if they were caught in time. Mommy was worried about me and was wondering how long I would be in theatre for. After about twenty minutes I was wheeled out of the theatre and back to the ward. Mommy and Daddy were called to the ward and waited with me until I woke up.

Oh no!

I felt sleepy when I woke up and went back to sleep. A little bit later I woke up again. I was confused because I was in a different room. Sr Susan came in the ward, asked me how I felt and gave me a big Winnie the Pooh. He was mine forever.

She told me I could go home when I felt better and had to come back on Monday for a Bone Scan and a C.A.T. scan to see if the cancer had spread anywhere else. They would also tell me what kind of cancer I had.

That weekend was a horrible one, Mommy and Daddy were very upset. We got many phone calls from friends and family and we did not know what to tell them because we did not know what was going to happen. We got a lot of letters and flowers from friends and family, saying good luck, and we miss you. I got a lovely card and present from my teacher. On the cover it said "To Someone Special."

> Dearest Sarah
>
> I've been thinking a lot about you!! Try keeping a "Journal scrapbook" of all your past, present and future experiences.
>
> Remember I love you very much!!

She gave me a scrapbook as a present. I also got another beautiful card from my principal with a huge bunch of flowers.

On Monday the 3rd of November 2003, we went back to the Oncology ward at the hospital. A lady doctor, Dr Janine came and introduced herself. She gave us the results of the biopsy.

I had Ewing's Sarcoma, a rare kind of cancer that normally affects children between seven and eighteen years. She explained that my treatment would consist of chemotherapy, an operation to remove the tumour and radiation. Then she gave me some bad news. She explained that I wasn't allowed to go to school until the treatment was over. I asked her how long that would be and she said my treatment would last about a year.

I was not allowed to visit any of my friends and they were not allowed to visit me. I looked at Dr Janine with wide eyes, she was full of bad news. She explained that my blood counts would get very low with the chemo and that would increase my chance of getting an infection. If I was in contact with somebody who was sick, my body would not be able to fight off the infection, and I would get sick. She also said that I was not allowed to eat any takeaway's, reheated foods, no biltong (dried meat) or yoghurt as these contained bacteria and might make me sick. Everything I ate had to be cooked properly.

I wasn't allowed to walk down Hospital Street. That was the fifth floor of the Joburg Gen where hundreds of people walked to their clinics. She said there were many bugs there that I could easily pick up and get really sick. She told us to walk across the sixth floor instead where there were less people. She also told my parents that I would be having thirteen blocks of chemo, each block would last for three days. After three weeks if my blood counts were good enough, I would get the next block of chemo. She said the treatment was very aggressive, because Ewing's Sarcoma was very aggressive. She explained that a lot of people do not come back to finish all their treatment and often their cancer came back. She told us we had to finish all the treatment otherwise I could die. This doctor was very clever and seemed to know everything about cancer. I was a bit scared of her because she looked quite strict.

She took me to the ward and told me to get onto a bed. She asked me for my arm and quickly put a needle in my vein. I screamed. It was so sore. My hand hurt! She connected me to a drip with a bag of watery stuff that dripped slowly into my vein. Then she left the room.

After a while I needed a wee, so Mommy helped me to the bathroom, she joked with me that I had to bring my "drip dog" for a walk. I giggled, it was time Mommy joked again. My drip dog was a bit difficult to walk. His wheels got stuck on the bed's wheels and Mommy had to help me. When I came back from the bathroom, I climbed back on my bed. After a while the nurses came in and wheeled me downstairs to the in-patient unit in Ward 286 on the eighth floor.

Sr Susan came with us and showed us around the ward and introduced us to some kids in the ward. She explained that some of the kids were given chemo for a few hours and could then go home, depending on their type of cancer. I asked her if this would happen to me, but she said that my type of cancer was vicious and I had to have very strong chemo to kill it off. She explained that each of my chemo blocks would last for three days, then if I was well enough after that I would be allowed to go home. She showed us the kitchen and the bathrooms and explained that no children were allowed to visit any of the cancer kids. She explained that because normal kids went to school and were in contact with lots of people, they could carry bugs that could make the cancer kids very sick. If a cancer kid's blood count was low, he would pick up an infection and possibly die from it. The ward was clean and I was happy to see that there was a bed for Mommy in my room. We unpacked our clothes in the cupboard.

Oh no!

I was bored and asked Mommy if we could go for a walk. She agreed and we walked out of the ward and down a long passage. I thought it was really fun to run and hold onto my drip, skiing down the corridors. As I swung around the corner, I accidentally crashed into the wall and my drip machine fell off its holder and cut the side of my face. I thought it was funny. Mommy was also laughing. We went back to the ward with blood dripping down my face while Mommy carried the drip box. As we walked into the ward the nurses asked us where we had been. They were cross and told me to stay in bed and not walk around. They told Mommy that I was not allowed out the ward at all. Dr Janine came in a little later to check on us and told Mommy that the stuff in the drip was to protect my kidneys before they started chemo. She asked me what had happened to my face, she was not happy and told me that I had to stay inside the ward.

Later that afternoon Daddy and Michelle came to visit, they laughed when we told them about the cut on my face. When they left, I really wanted to go home with them. That night when I wanted to sleep, my drip kept blocking. It beeped every time it blocked, and I would wake up instantly. The nurses walked in and out of my room often to fix my drip. In the middle of the night one of the nurses said, "Oh no we have to take your drip out, it's blocked again." I was scared. I did not know what she was going to do and started crying. I grabbed Mommy's hand and squeezed it hard. I screamed as I felt the needle touch my hand. The nurse said, "Shoosh, you will wake the others, they are sleeping."

I ignored her and carried on screaming. It was very sore, I was starting to hate needles and drips. When she had finished, I fell asleep crying, I missed home, I missed Daddy and Michelle, I knew I always fought with her but I missed her now and promised myself I would never fight with her again. I also missed my dogs Timmy, Slinky and Dusty, and my two cats, Whisper and Rambo. All I wanted to do was go home, see my family and have no big needles in my hand.

The next day was Tuesday. When I woke up the sun was shining brightly in my eyes. I had to go downstairs for a Bone Scan, I was scared because I did not know what they were going to do to me. Mommy held my hand all the time while the nurse pushed my bed into the lift. A nurse told me to move onto another bed with a big machine above it that would scan my body. She started the machine, it moved down towards me, I had to lie very still. The machine kept on coming closer and closer.

"Mommy, it's gonna squish me, stop it!" I started crying.

Oh no!

The nurse told me not to worry, that it had to come down close to my body so that it could scan my bones and that it was nearly all over. The machine stopped just on the top of my body and a doctor was looking at a computer screen. He explained to Mommy that this machine was scanning all the bones in my body, looking for cancer. He said that my kind of cancer spreads to the bones very quickly. He showed Mommy that none of my bones had any cancer in them and that we are lucky to have come in for treatment so soon.

He explained that Ewing's Sarcoma moves into the bones and lungs quickly and if you do not catch it in time, you can die. Mommy was happy that my cancer was only in the muscles in my leg and had not spread anywhere. When the scan was finished, the nurse pushed my drip away so that I could get off the machine but the wheels of my drip dog had hooked on something on the floor and the drip machine fell on the floor and broke. I thought it was funny and started laughing. Mommy was giggling as well and the nurse quickly picked up the drip and put it back together again.

After that I went for a C.A.T. scan to see which muscles were affected by the tumour. We went into a different room and I was put in another big machine. This machine did not move close to me and it wasn't sore.

Mommy stayed next to me and had to wear a lead apron so that the radiation from the scanner did not affect her. When it was over, the nurse explained to us that the tumour had affected some muscles on the front of my thigh. We went back to the ward where Mommy read a story to me and I fell asleep. It had been a busy day.

On Wednesday fifth November my first chemo block started. I remember sitting on my hospital bed playing Barbies with Mommy. A nurse came in and changed the bag on the drip, this was my first bag of chemo. She gave Mommy a brown paper bag in case I vomited and showed Mommy where to get more in case I needed them. I watched it drip slowly and Mommy was wondering what kind of reaction I would have. The doctors had told her that I would vomit, feel nauseous, have mouth ulcers and that my hair might fall out. Now I understood why so many kids there had no hair. I wondered what I would look like with no hair and if I would be bald forever. That was a scary thought.

That first bag of chemo only took about an hour and I was feeling fine. Mommy and I were laughing and joking when the nurse walked in with the next bag. This nurse chatted a lot to my mom and told her all about ward life and what to expect. She told us that the main thing was to be positive and that we mustn't worry because I would be fine.

When the second bag of chemo was finished, Mommy went and called a nurse. She took the empty bag off the drip and put on a third bag. This one was terrible, I didn't feel well at all and felt like vomiting. I told Mommy and she quickly gave me the brown paper bag. Soon the bag was full and Mommy quickly got another but she was too late - I had messed on the sheets. Yuck! My eyes were watering and my hair kept on falling in my face. Soon I had filled four paper bags full of vomit! My sheets, pillow and pyjamas had puke on them, it smelt terrible.

Mommy went and asked the nurse for clean sheets. The nurse showed her where to get clean sheets if I needed more. Mommy helped me off the bed and sat me in a chair next to my bed. She helped me change out of my pyjamas and then she changed the sheets. I felt horrible and I climbed back onto the bed and fell asleep.

Later on, a nurse came into my ward and gave me some red mouthwash. She told me to rinse my mouth often to stop mouth ulcers from forming. I got off the bed, pushed my drip dog to the basin and rinsed my mouth. It tasted and smelt disgusting. Everything was starting to smell funny. When that bag of chemo was finished I felt a little bit better and played Barbies with Mommy. I was tired and fell asleep again.

I hated the drip, it hurt me, it was always blocking or the needle bent and the nurses had to keep on taking it out and putting it back again, it was sore. I had another bag of chemo and vomited even more, I was using up many paper bags. All I wanted to eat was bacon. Mommy phoned Daddy and asked him to bring me some bacon biscuits when he visited us that night. I could not wait for him and Michelle to visit. When they eventually came, I ate nearly the whole box of biscuits before they left. I was sad when they went home.

On Friday seventh November Dr Janine came to check on me; she was happy with my progress and said I could go home.

The nurses came to take the drip out but before they did, Mommy told me not to scream and to concentrate on the fact that we were going home. But I couldn't, it was too sore and I screamed and screamed. I was not feeling very well, but happy to be going home. As we climbed into the car I told Mommy that I felt like vomiting. She had brought a paper bag with her in case I vomited. On the way home, I told Mommy to stop the car because I was going to vomit. We stopped on the side of the road and Mommy had to hold my hair out of the way while I vomited on the pavement. Many people who were driving past, slowed down to look at me. When I got home I was very tired and slept. The dogs all came to lie with me, I was happy to be home.

The next Thursday I had to go back to the hospital for a check-up. We had to go to Hospital Street for a finger prick test. I did not know what they were going to do, Mommy told me they had to test my blood to see what the chemo was doing to my blood count. We met Sr Belinda, she was very kind and patient. There were two kids who had to have their fingers pricked before me. I looked around the room at all the toys and books. Everything was so bright and colourful. I asked Mommy if I could play with some toy dinosaurs. I was having fun and then Sr Belinda called me, it was my turn. Mommy came with me to Sr Belinda's table and I sat on her lap. Sr Belinda chatted to me and asked me what kind of cancer I had, but all I could think about was this long needle going into my finger.

I started wiggling on Mommy's lap but Sr Belinda helped Mommy to hold my hand tightly. I screamed, but it was over quickly and Sr Belinda put a plaster on my finger and gave me a sweet. She smiled kindly at us and told Mommy that many of the kids were scared in the beginning and that I would soon get used to it. I did not think I could ever get used to THAT. She told us to go upstairs to the ninth floor for a checkup. As I walked down the long corridors, I saw Mommy was crying. I told her that I was fine.

We both cheered up when we were upstairs. Sr Susan was there to greet us again and took me to the room full of toys, books and puzzles. She asked me what I wanted to do. I chose a puzzle and took it to the waiting room. Some CHOC volunteers were there busily baking biscuits with some of the other kids. They asked me if I wanted to join in. It looked like fun. Everybody was so friendly and chatted to me. I made friends with a boy called Ben. He had leukaemia and was not well at all. His mom chatted to us for a long time.

After a while Dr Janine called me for my checkup. First they weighed me, I was twenty kilograms. Then they measured me, I was 1.22m. Then I went into Dr Janine's office. It was also brightly painted and had a few toys on her desk. She checked my leg, pushed my tummy, looked in my ears and throat and then sat down at her desk. She explained to Mommy that I would be getting my next bag of chemo soon, if my blood counts were good enough. She said sometimes the chemo catches the hair cycle in the wrong place and then your hair falls out, but if it does not then you do not lose your hair. She said that some kids do not lose their hair. Mommy did not like bald kids. Dr Janine was happy with me, but told me not to fight with the nurses when they put up a drip. I did not think she had ever had a drip put in her, because she would have known my pain. Maybe Dr Janine was really tough and drips didn't hurt her. Then we went home, Mommy and I sang songs in the car.

Mommy was lucky that she was able to take time off work to take me for my checkups. At home we had a lady looking after me. She really wanted to be a nurse, but never had the money to study. She was sweet and looked after me well. She helped me with my homework and helped Mommy around the house.

Mommy and Daddy took me for a haircut. They knew that my hair would be falling out, so they wanted to cut it short. I loved my new hairstyle, it was so much easier to wash.

One day I was sitting in the lounge colouring in. I loved colouring in and used lots of different coloured crayons. I ran my fingers through my hair and was shocked to find a whole lot of it in my hand. As I got up, another lot of hair fell on the floor. I ran into my room and looked in the mirror, my hair was looking a little bit patchy. I was too scared to touch it, in case more fell out. Soon Mommy would be home from work, I could not wait to show her what was happening. I waited at the door and as she opened it, I didn't even greet her, I just said, "Mommy look! My hair is falling out!"

Mommy was shocked and quietly turned away and went into the bathroom and burst into tears. She had hoped that my hair would not fall out. Later that afternoon when I was in the bath my Ouma (granny) came to visit. I heard Daddy's car arrive and looked down at the bath water. There was hair everywhere, I shouted for Mommy. She came into the bathroom with Ouma and was shocked. I could see the tears in her eyes, but Ouma laughed and said that I would look quite funny without hair. Michelle came into the bathroom to see what was going on. She told me not to rub my hair with the towel in case some more hair fell out.

The next morning I woke up and looked at my pillow. There was hair everywhere. Mommy had to vacuum my pillows, sheet, duvet and even my teddy bears. Mommy was shocked as she thought my hair would fall out slowly over the next couple of weeks, but I only had about half a head of hair left.

The next day was Saturday and Daddy told me that

Oh no!

he wanted to shave my hair off because I looked even more patchy. We shaved our heads together, it felt good to know I was not the only bald one, I loved feeling Daddy's smooth head, then mine. I was happy that I didn't look so patchy but I felt weird. I knew that people would stare at me. Over the next few weeks I was given a couple of beanies and caps to wear. They all made my head itch and I decided not to wear them.

I remember going to the shops and having lots of people stop and stare at me. It did not bother me at all, if they wanted to look, they could.

On Wednesday twenty-sixth November, I had to go back to hospital for another block of chemo. I hated the 'finger prick' and wouldn't let Sr Belinda take blood, it was way too sore. I didn't even want to go into her room. Sr Belinda explained that she would be really quick and that I must not scream and fight. I couldn't help it, I was just so scared. Eventually she gave up and the nurses had to take blood from my arm in the ward upstairs. Three nurses had to hold me down, I kicked and screamed and hated every minute of it. A little later they started a drip with chemo. I stayed in the day ward until three p.m.

Then they took me downstairs to the proper ward. I did not mind staying in hospital because Mommy read

Spunky

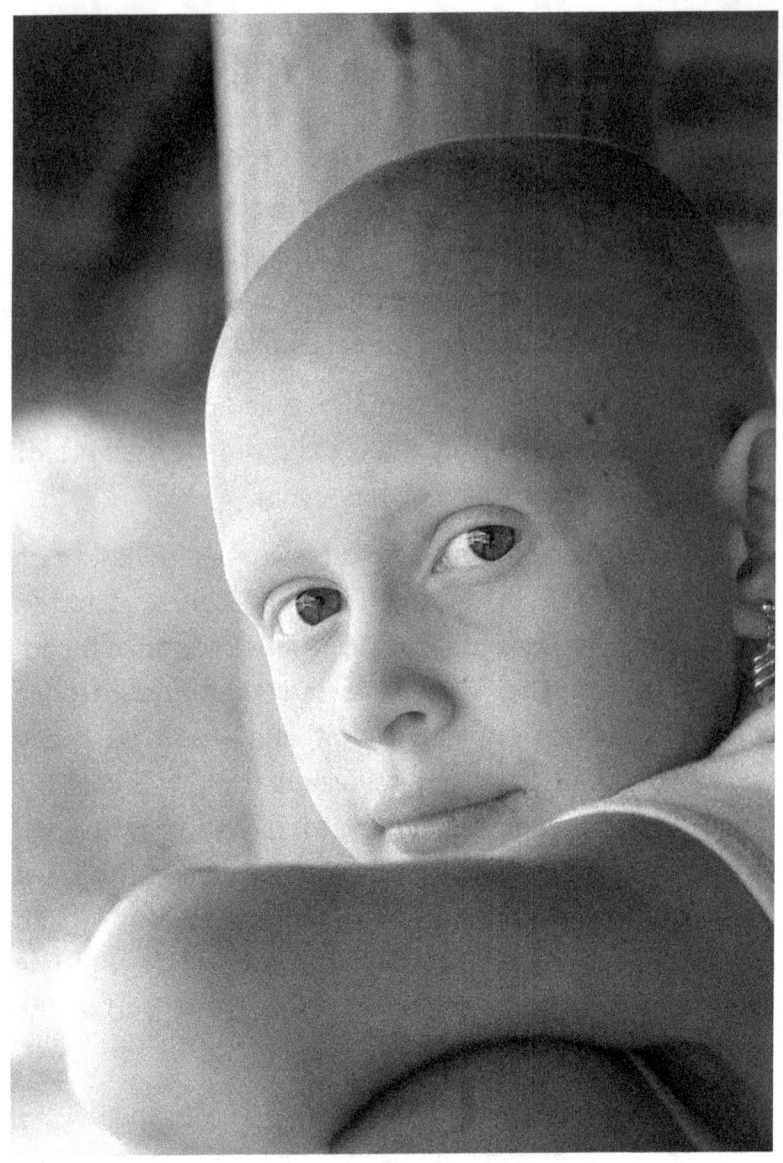

Me without hair

me many stories and played games with me. Then we had some surprise visitors, some clowns came into my ward! They played lots of magic tricks and one small clown rode his little scooter around the ward. He was just a little bit taller than I was. I wished that I could also ride on his scooter. The clowns visited all the children in the ward. Their magic tricks were the best and I could not understand how they could make a piece of string longer and longer and longer. I kept asking them how they did their tricks, but they just smiled and winked at me.

Ben was in the ward next to me. He had an infection and had to stay in hospital until it cleared. He wasn't allowed any visitors. He was supposed to get his next block of chemo but had to wait until his infection cleared. His mom was worried about him and spoke to Mommy for a long time in the passage.

My drip kept on giving trouble. I did not feel so sick with this lot of chemo and vomited less than last time. Andrea, the counsellor came to see me. She spoke to Mommy about my problem with the drip, she said she could help me because I should not be fighting with the nurses every time they needed to put up a drip. She did not understand how sore it was. Just after she left, the drip's needle bent AGAIN. A nurse took me into a small operating theatre in the centre of the ward.

Four nurses came in and held me down while they put the drip back in my hand. Mommy was talking to me all the time, telling me not to fight and to keep still. I couldn't help myself, I starting kicking and screaming. The one nurse leaned over me and I bit her. I was not a good patient and the nurses did not like me either. I really wanted to go home.

On Friday twenty-eighth November Andrea came to talk to me again. I met her puppet, a dog called Bruno and then we had to go downstairs to the finger prick room. I was so scared that I would have my finger pricked again. Sr Belinda was there with a big smile on her face. She asked me how I was, I did not want to be there and was grumpy. I wiped away my tears. Andrea explained that they had to do a finger prick on me every time I came to the hospital to check my blood count. She told me that only Bruno was going to get his finger pricked that day, not me. I was relieved. She said that he could have a sweet afterwards if he was good.

"But, Bruno can't eat!" I mumbled.

"Then if you and Bruno are good, you can have both of them!" she said.

Then she sat Bruno on her lap and pricked his finger. Andrea told me that it's okay to be scared, but not to fight.

Oh no!

She showed me what I looked like through Bruno, she made him kick and scream just like I did, it was actually very funny, to see a puppet kick and scream.

Andrea asked me why I was so scared and I told her that I thought there was a very big needle inside the machine that would go all the way up my finger. Then Sr Belinda opened up the finger prick machine to show me the size of the needle. It was tiny, I was amazed as they both told me that I must not be scared anymore and that it was much easier and quicker to take blood from somebody who sits still and doesn't fight. Then Andrea took me to the adult section and showed me around. These patients also had to have their fingers pricked.

On Monday the first of December I had to see Andrea again. She took me back into Sr Belinda's room and I watched the other children having their fingers pricked. I was feeling better about finger pricks when I saw that there were other kids going through the same thing. Some of them cried a little bit and others were good and sat still. I told myself that I had to be strong and not fight anymore. Sr Belinda explained that it was much easier for her if I sat still as she could work quickly. Daddy took me for a finger prick on Thursday fourth December. I was scared but I decided not to fight. I was proud of myself for not screaming.

Then we went upstairs and Dr Janine checked me. She said the chemo had shrunk the tumour a lot, which was good news. But my blood count was low, which was bad news. I was not allowed to visit anybody in case I got sick, not even Roxy, my best friend. I missed her so much.

A week later Daddy took me for another finger prick and check-up. Dr Janine told him that they were going to operate to take the tumour out. I was scared and started crying. She told Daddy that my blood count was up which meant that my body was strong enough for the operation.

Ghosty-Ghosty

I had to be at the hospital before seven a.m. on Monday fifteenth December 2003 for my operation. A nurse came into my ward and gave me a long gown to put on. Mommy helped me change out of my pyjamas and into the gown. It was too big for me and reached all the way to the floor. I giggled and told Mommy that now I could play ghosty-ghosty. We were laughing when the nurses came to take me to theatre. They said that I was first on the theatre list that morning, so I had to hurry. I did not enjoy that ride, they pushed me down the corridor quickly and all the lights on the ceiling made me dizzy. As we got out of the lift I saw that Mommy was crying and trying to wipe her tears away. I asked her what was wrong. She said she was really worried about me.

"But Mommy, you mustn't worry about me, I will be fine," I said with a big smile on my face. I taught my mom a big lesson that day. The only way to get through all of this was by being positive. Nothing could work properly if you are negative.

The operating theatre was small. Mommy was chatting to the surgeons and asked if she could stay with me and watch the operation. They told her that tumours in the leg had a lot of blood vessels and that the operation would be very bloody and messy. They told her to rather go upstairs and have a cup of coffee. Then Mommy asked them if they could keep a piece of the tumour to show her. They said they would. Then they put a mask on my face and Mommy kissed my cheek, her tears dripped on to my forehead. Again, the doctor told me to count to ten. While I was counting, I was wondering if he knew how to count for himself and then everything went black.

The operation took a long time. Then I was wheeled back into the ward. The surgeons spoke to Mommy while I was sleeping. They had to cut out a big tumour, which measured 8cm x 12cm. The tumour was in the muscles in my thigh and ran across the main nerve in my leg. If they had cut out the whole tumour, they would have cut the nerve and I would be paralysed and would never be able to walk again. So instead they cut on either side of the nerve, but this meant that some cancer cells were left behind. They said that the rest of the blocks of chemo and the radiation would kill off those left over cancer cells. They explained to Mommy that because the tumour was so big, they had to cut out nearly all the muscles in the front of my thigh. This meant that I would have to learn how to walk again. I woke up a few times and then went back to sleep. I was really thirsty.

Mommy was next to me and so I asked her for some water. She gave me a little bit of water to drink but suddenly I vomited it all out. The nurse came in and was cross with Mommy for giving me water. She said Mommy should have waited a while first. She helped clean me up and I went back to sleep.

The next day I was still very sleepy. I had small sips of water but slept most of the day. I had a Portavac in my leg to drain the wound. They had also put a Hickman line in my chest. This was a tube going into the vein in my heart so that they would not need to put drips in my hand anymore. I was so glad. I really hated those drips that always blocked. I thought the nurses would be happy that they would not have to fight with me anymore. Ben's mom popped into my ward to see how I was doing. Poor Ben was back in for his next block of chemo.

On Wednesday seventeenth December I was still on a drip and slept all day. I wondered what Mommy did while I was sleeping?

The next day I woke up starving. I ate two bowls of Fruit Loops, watched TV, played Barbies and Uno with Mommy. I had many visitors that day, they all came from different companies. They visited every child in the ward and gave us many Christmas presents.

Four soccer players from Orlando Pirates visited and I had my photo taken with them. They gave me cool drink and sweets. Then Sr Susan came into the ward and introduced me to a man who had also had a Ewing's Sarcoma when he was thirteen years old. His tumour was in his hip and because the doctor's did not know what it was, it grew to be the size of a soccer ball. His cancer spread to his thighbone so he had had three hip replacements. Now he was completely clear of cancer. He was brave and I wanted to be like him and be clear of cancer too. This was the first person I had met who had the same kind of cancer as me. Most of the other kids in the ward had leukaemia or brain tumours. Their treatment was different to mine.

Then the nurses came in to take out my Portavac. I did not want them to touch me and told them that I wanted to take it out myself. They knew me by now and how much I could fight, so they showed me what to do. Then they had to flush out my Hickman line. First they took the plaster off my chest and unravelled the plastic tube, which was stitched on to me. Then they cleaned it, curled up the pipe and covered it with a new plaster. I tried so hard not to fight and scream, but I ended up crying. The nurse told me that I wasn't allowed to get the plaster wet. I had to be very careful when I washed and had to keep the area clean so that it would not get infected.

I could not walk or get out of bed. Every time I needed a wee, I had to use a bed pan. Mommy found out where they kept the bed pans so that she didn't have to keep on calling the nurse when I needed one.

It was then that I heard a lot of excitement from the kids down the corridor in the other wards and I wondered what was going on. I wished I could get out of bed and go and see what was happening. Mommy went to look and told me that the actors from the pantomime **Jack and the Beanstalk** had come to visit.

They wore pretty costumes and visited every kid in the ward. My ward was right at the end of the passage and I could not wait for them to come and visit me. A few minutes later they popped into my ward. Two of the actresses sat on my bed and spent a long time chatting to me while the rest of them visited the next ward. When they eventually left, they gave me complimentary tickets to see their show and told me to come backstage when the show was over. They gave me their phone numbers and told me to phone them. I was so excited to watch the show and wondered how I was going to walk. Mommy told me that she would get a wheelchair and some crutches.

The next day a nurse brought me a wheelchair. It was a small kid's size and was bright red. Mommy said she was happy I did not weigh much because she had to pick me up and put me in it. I could not stand or walk but soon I was whizzing around the ward. I met another little girl who was also in a wheelchair. The nurse told Mommy that she also had Ewing's Sarcoma but hers was in her spine. She couldn't walk properly and had been in a wheelchair for a while.

Many other famous people who were on TV or were actors visited the cancer ward over Christmas time. They all sat on my bed and asked me what had happened to me. I was lucky to meet so many people. Most of them brought me presents or sweets.

On Friday nineteenth December one of the doctors gave me some good news. She said I could start walking. Mommy and I were excited and I asked her to put my slippers on and help me off my bed so that I could stand again. I was so excited, but when I put my feet on the floor, I just collapsed. I was surprised and looked at Mommy. Her eyes were wide with worry, she did not expect me to be so weak. She picked me up and put me back on the bed again.

Later when the doctor came to check on me, she had another lady with her. She introduced me to her and told me that this lady was a Physiotherapist and she would help me to learn how to walk again. She explained that they had cut out nearly all the muscles in the front of my thigh and that I would have to learn how to walk again. They helped me out of bed and held me up while I tried to stand. It felt strange to be on my feet after being in bed for so long. Then they told me to try and walk just a few steps. I couldn't even walk to the door which was near my bed.

The Physio explained that it would take a while and that I would slowly build up enough strength to walk farther and farther. It felt so strange because my brain wanted to walk and run, but my body could not. I turned around and struggled to walk another few steps. I was really tired and she picked me up and put me in bed again. Later on that day she took me for another slow walk. She also gave me exercises to do in my bed. These made me tired.

The next day the Physio came and I took another few steps with her. She told me to do my exercises every day. Before she left she told Mommy that I must try and walk a few times every day with somebody holding me up. After lunch, I asked Mommy to take me for a walk. I really wanted to reach the door, but I could not. My leg was too sore. Later that afternoon I walked around really slowly with Mommy holding me again. This time I made it to the door I stood for a while and then tried to walk back to my bed. I was exhausted and could not make it, so Mommy carried me back to my bed. Later that afternoon I did my exercises in bed.

That evening Mommy went home and Daddy stayed with me for the weekend, but it was a bit boring because Daddy didn't play as many games with me. Each day I walked a little bit more and was soon able to walk to the door and back.

On Sunday twenty-first December I was getting stronger and was starting to walk a few steps on my own. Mommy was happy to see my progress when she came back in the evening. She and Daddy chatted for a while and then Daddy went home. He was glad to go home to a comfortable bed.

Early on Monday morning the doctor visited me. He explained that the muscles that they had cut out, cannot regrow. Some other stuff called fibrous tissue grows in its place. This is not elastic like muscle and can snap easily so I was not allowed to run or jump for a long time. I wasn't really bothered about this and just wanted to be home for Christmas.

Lots of people visited me, mostly friends and family, but also a lot of strangers who walked around the ward giving the kids sweets and cake. The CHOC volunteers were always in the ward, reading stories to the kids or sitting on their beds chatting. I had made friends with a lot of them. They were all holding thumbs that I would be able to go home for Christmas.

I had no feeling above my knee, it was weird, because when you rub your leg, you are supposed to feel it, it was so strange. The surgeon came to check on me and I asked him about this funny feeling. He explained that he had to cut smaller nerves in my leg and that the feeling would not ever come back. I was just so happy to be walking again. I still was not able to walk far or very quickly, but I knew I would get stronger.

I was really looking forward to seeing Uncle Andrew for Christmas. Uncle Andrew was my mom's brother. He was a Marine Engineer and worked on ships. He lived in Cape Town and worked off the coast of Angola. When he came home, he would fly to us for a visit. We did not see him often, but when we did it was so exciting.

On Christmas Eve most of the children in the ward were sent home for Christmas. I was really hoping to be one of them and then Dr Moore, one of the oncologists came into my ward and told me that I could go home. Mommy spoke to him about borrowing one of the small wheelchairs. He said we could take it home and use it for as long as I needed it.

Spunky

Mommy picked me up and put me in the wheelchair while she packed my clothes. I wheeled myself out of the ward, it was quite hard and my arms ached. I soon discovered that I could do wheelies on it. Mommy caught me and told me to stop. Then she told me to wait upstairs in the ward, while she took our bags, duvets and pillows down to the car. Then she came back for me and my new red wheels. I couldn't wait to get home to eat some tomatoes. I had been craving them.

At home the dogs and cats were so happy to see me. I asked Mommy to fetch me a tomato from the fridge. When I had finished it, I asked her for another one and then another one. Soon I had finished a whole bag all on my own. Mommy organized a pair of crutches for me. They were quite difficult to walk with in the beginning but I soon got used to them. If I used them for a long time, my hands got sore.

We fetched Uncle Andrew from the airport and he stayed with us for Christmas. Mommy and Michelle did last minute Christmas shopping. Mommy had been in hospital with me and had not had a chance to buy all the presents in time. That night I couldn't sleep and was so excited to see what was in the presents under the Christmas tree. It was a battle not being able to walk properly and I had to call Mommy a few times in the middle of the night for a wee. Luckily I was very light and Mommy did not have a problem picking me up.

The next morning I was up early. We all waited eagerly for Daddy to play Father Christmas and hand out the Christmas presents. I was so happy to be home. We had a lovely day and Michelle and I got many presents. Uncle Andrew gave me a whole case of custard. He had always called me the 'Custard Monster' because I love it so much.

On Sunday twenty-eighth December it was Uncle Andrew's fortieth Birthday. We had a braai (barbeque) in the afternoon and invited some of our family to the party. It was not a big party, but Uncle Andrew enjoyed it.

I was getting used to walking on crutches and could move around quickly. I battled to carry things and had to ask for help all the time. But it was still better than being in hospital. A few days later we took Uncle Andrew to the airport and he flew home to Cape Town.

I was really looking forward to the **Jack and the Beanstalk** show, even though I battled a bit with my crutches. Daddy, Mommy, Michelle and I watched the show, sitting really close to the stage so we could see everything. The costumes were beautiful and the show was excellent.

Afterwards we were allowed to go back stage. All the cast members were waiting for me and as I opened the backstage door they starting cheering. I spent a long time chatting to them. They took me into their change rooms to see their cupboards full of clothes. I swapped phone numbers with a lot of the actresses and have stayed in contact with them. All the actors and actresses wrote messages for me in my autograph book, wishing me good luck with the rest of my treatment.

Burnt

Early in 2004 I was booked in for chemo again. This time I vomited even more. I didn't feel like eating or drinking anything and everything tasted and smelled strange. Mommy's food smelled funny and I told her not to eat it in the ward because it made me feel worse. I started getting 'shocking pains' in my leg, when my leg would twitch on its own. One of the Oncologists came to check on me, I told her about my leg jumping. She said it was a good sign because the nerves in my leg were slowly growing back together. She said that the feeling in my leg would slowly come back in places. She also said that we had to start radiation. I did not know what she was talking about and asked Mommy later. She didn't know either. I just hoped it did not mean needles and drips again.

Ben was back in hospital again. He kept on getting infections and was not well at all. He was back in the isolation ward where nobody was allowed to visit him.

We had to go to the Hillbrow Hospital for radiation. All the departments in this hospital had closed down, only the Radiation Department was still there. It was a dirty hospital and smelled bad, but the staff were friendly.

I was not sure what they were going to do to me. First I had to go to the Mould Room where I had to lie on a table on two black plastic bags. The doctor poured some liquid in one of the bags and very quickly poured something else in the other bag. There the two liquids mixed together and started to rise against me. I had to keep very still – it was hard because this mixture was hot. It was also difficult because I could not keep my bad leg in the same position for a long time. When it had set, they lifted me out of the mould.

I had to come back the next day because there was lots to do before they could start the radiation. They did another C.A.T. scan – I was a bit scared because this hospital was really old and the machine made funny noises. Mommy stayed with me and the doctor told her to wear a heavy lead apron. Then they took me to a Simulation Room. It was dark in there and there was a big machine in the middle of the room.

They brought in my mould, put it on a table and picked me up to lie in it and then they had to tattoo me. They had to do this so that they could line up the radiation machine properly and make sure that they would not radiate in the wrong places. They started the first tattoo on the top of my thigh. It was very, very sore and I screamed and screamed. The doctor spoke to my mom and told her that I needed to be sedated for them to carry on. So I got out of my mould and went to the doctor's room down the passage. I was given some medicine and we went to the waiting room. I sat on Mommy's lap and soon got very, very sleepy. Mommy carried me back into the Simulation Room where they finished tattooing my legs and tummy. I was very drowsy when they did this and cried a lot. After that I was allowed to go home. I fell asleep in the back of the car.

The next day we had to go back to the Hillbrow Hospital again. The doctors said my mould was not right and they had to redo it again. This time I knew what they were going to do, so I wasn't scared. I was wearing an open backed shirt and the mixture was very hot when I lay down on the plastic bags. One of the nurses put some roller towel between the black plastic bags and my skin, which felt better.

After that I had to go back into the Simulation Room. I was so scared that they were going to tattoo me again, but the doctor told me that there was not going to be any more pain. Now I had to lie in the mould again and they had to line up the red laser beams on the mould. I had to keep still while the doctors measured lots of things. Then they took me into the radiation room to look around. There was a thick steel door before we went in – so the radiation cannot come out of the room because it is very dangerous. On the way home Mommy and I talked about radiation. She didn't know anybody who had had radiation before.

The next week I had to go to the Joburg Gen for another finger prick and a checkup. Everything was fine. I was proud of myself for not fighting or screaming. One of the nurses noticed that I behaved better and she smiled at me and told me she was happy that I was not giving them a hard time anymore.

On the twenty-eighth of January the preparation for radiation was finished and now they could start. I had to take off my jeans, socks and takkies (sandshoes). They picked me up to put me in my mould on the table. Then they had to line up the laser beams again. The nurse told me to fold my arms across my chest. The machine moved to the right position making a strange noise when it turned. They told me to keep still until they came back. Mommy went out of the room and watched me from the other room on the computer screen. I had radiation for one minute and then all the doctors and nurses came back into the room. They gave me a white card, which had to be signed every day when they had finished. I had to come back every day for twenty-five sessions of radiation not including weekends.

Burnt

The radiation didn't hurt at all. I met lots of people there and made friends quickly with the students. Once a week I had to go to Dr Coetzee for a check-up who was in charge of the Radiation Department. He checked my leg and was happy with my progress.

I also had to go to the Joburg Gen once a week for a finger prick and checkup with any of the Oncologists. I liked all the doctors, but Doctor Janine was still my favourite. It's weird, because even at school, I would like the strictest teacher who would still shout at me. The finger pricks were not so bad anymore and I didn't fight. I did not have any chemo while I was going through the radiation. After the check-up I went for radiation.

My radiation carried on every day until the ninth February. My skin on my leg was slowly starting to go dark brown. I was not allowed to bath with soap, use any creams, bubble bath or even dry my leg with a towel. I also wasn't allowed to wear any jeans or tight fitting clothes, which was a problem, because most of my pants were either jeans or were quite tight. Mommy found really loose fitting skirts, which were quite comfortable.

On the second February I had another check-up. Dr Janine checked my leg and was happy with me. Ben was in the waiting room. He had also had his finger pricked. I chatted to him for a long time. He told me that he had also hated fingerpicks in the beginning but that he had got used to them. He was tired of being in hospital and wished he was well, like his sisters.

A week later I found going to the toilet was sore. Mommy phoned the hospital and spoke to Dr Moore, one of the Oncologists. He said that I needed to come in and see him and bring in a urine sample because he thought I had an infection. I couldn't even manage to give him a few drops of wee and cried in pain. He gave me some antibiotics and we went home.

The next week I had another check-up at the Joburg Gen. Every day the pain was getting worse and worse. I could not sit flat on my bum, it was too sore. The skin on my bad leg started to get blisters and so did my tummy and my good leg. Dr Coetzee had a look and told me to use Gentian Violet. Mommy took me home and put some Gentian Violet on some cotton wool and told me to dab it on the bottom part of the blisters where it wasn't that sore. I screamed in pain and Mommy told me we should just leave it.

At the next check-up at the Joburg Gen Dr Janine decided to stop the radiation until my burns had healed. I was still very sore and could not even sit in the bath. She said that my skin and all the organs in that area had been burnt by the radiation. My skin was black and had big blisters. I asked Dr Janine if I would have these blisters when I was older, she said that they would disappear but there would be scarring which would eventually fade.

Miracles do happen

Two weeks later I had some good news. Two of my mom's friends had organized that I go to a local radio station to meet the **Rude Awakening** team. I loved Jeremy Mansfield and was so excited. I listened to them every morning and now I was going to meet them. We drove through to the studios, I tried not to think of the pain in my leg. When I got there everybody was excited to see me and give me a big hug. I went into a small studio where I sat on Jeremy's lap. Then the music stopped and he started talking to me about my cancer and my treatment. I was shy because I knew all my friends and family would be listening. I also chatted to Samantha Cowan who hosted the show with Jeremy.

After the radio show was over, we went to Sandton Square for some photos. My mom's friends wanted me to be on the cover of a magazine. I felt so special. We had chocolate milkshakes and I enjoyed chasing the birds in Sandton Square. There were many people there and they all stared at me. I was so used to people being rude about my bald head. They did not know what I had been through and probably didn't even know what cancer was.

Spunky

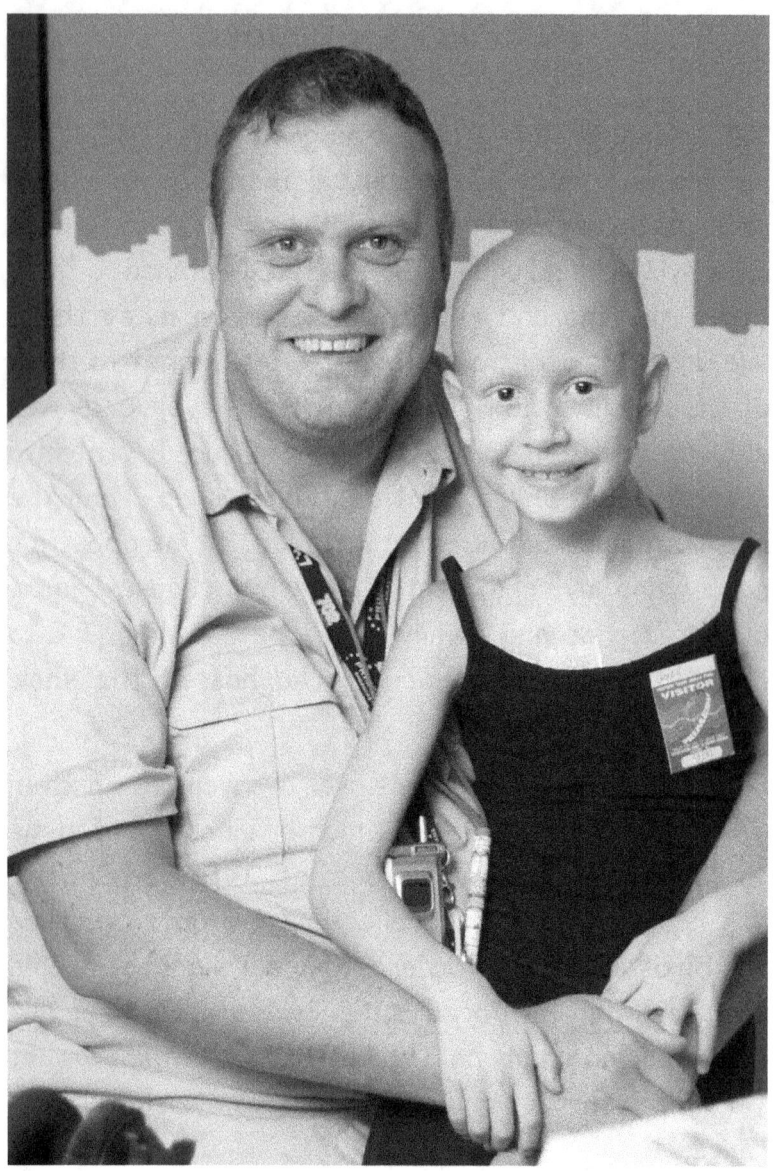

Jeremy Mansfield and me

Miracles do happen

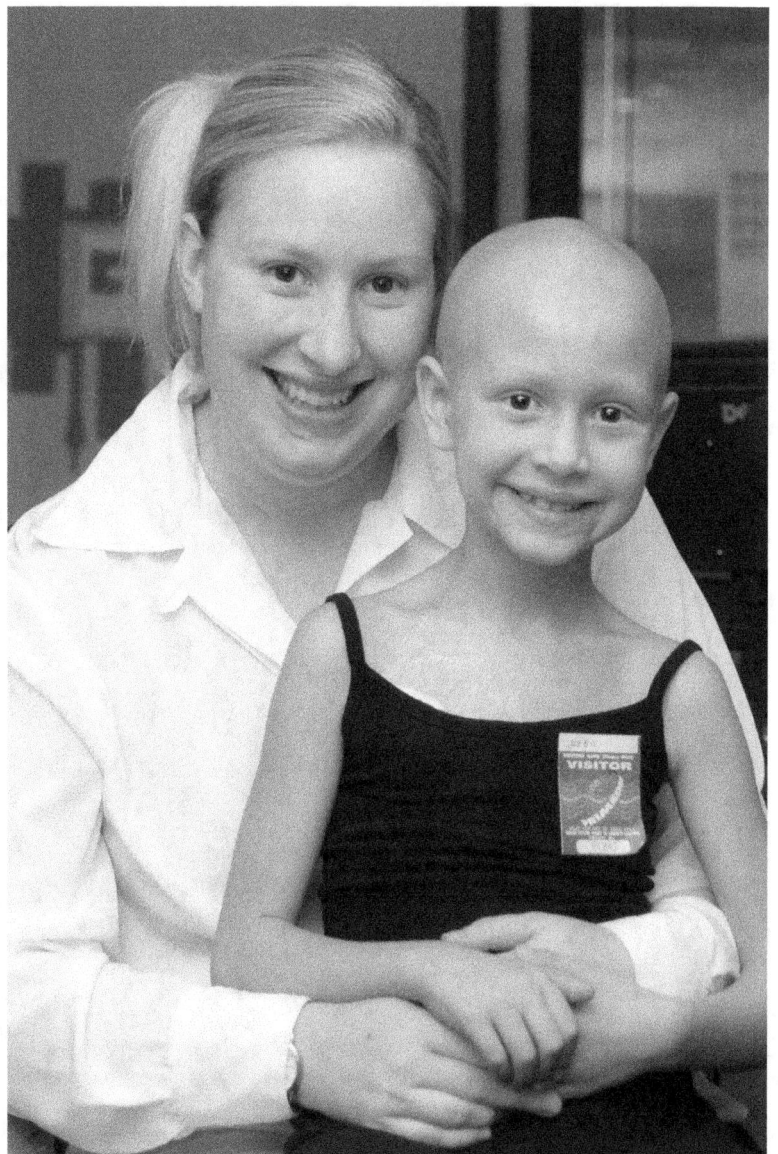

Samantha Cowan and me

Spunky

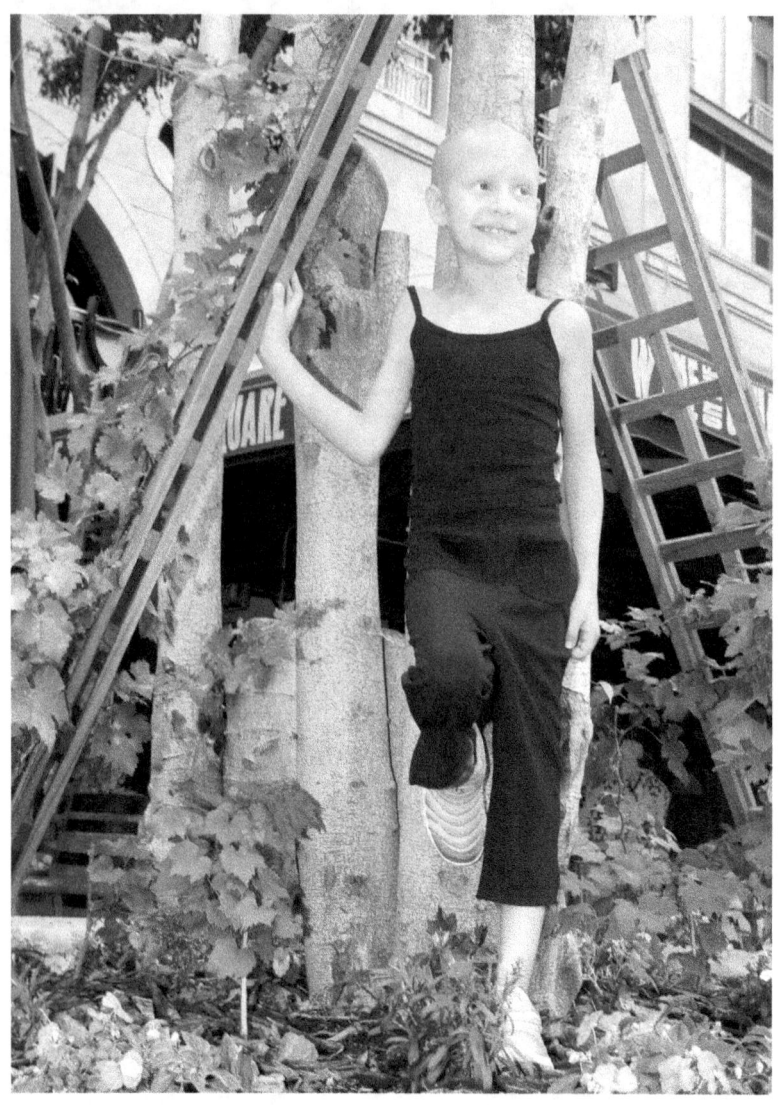

Me in Sandton Square

Miracles do happen

The next week I went back to the Joburg Gen for another check-up. There were some people in the ward who took a photo of me for another magazine. I was getting quite famous. When I was younger, I had always dreamed of being in a magazine. Every time we went for a check-up, Mommy looked for Ben and his mom. They seemed to live in hospital.

A week later Mommy's friends organised a huge party for me at a restaurant close to home. All the Grade two's (my class from the previous year) and that year's Grade threes were invited. I was so happy to see all my old friends and tried not to think of the burns on my leg. My new Grade three teacher and my old Grade two teacher were there. A lot of other people were there too, all giving me presents. I felt so special. One of Mommy's friends baked a chocolate teddy-bear cake and the restaurant gave all my friends yummy food. My actress friend from **Jack in the Beanstalk** was there too. She always made everything such fun.

Half way through the party, Daddy called me up in front of everybody and told me to turn around and close my eyes. Everybody was suddenly very quiet. I felt someone spin me around, to face the other way and everybody shouted, "Okay, open".

Spunky

I opened my eyes and there was Barbie. I loved Barbie and was so excited to see her. She also gave me presents and played games with my friends and me. It was a day I would never forget.

Then it was time to start radiation again. My burns had not really healed much but they had to carry on otherwise the cancer would regrow. I was scared, because I knew I would be burnt again. When we walked into the Radiation Department I met an old lady who was crying. Mommy went and spoke to her, she also had cancer and wanted to give up and not carry on with her treatment. She was very sad and said there was no point in carrying on, she said she was going to die anyway. I smiled at her and felt sorry for her. Then she started talking to me and asking me why I was there. I told her I also had cancer and that I was having radiation. She said I was brave and I told her that she must also be brave, carry on with her treatment, and never give up. She hugged me hard and told me I was very special. I was so happy to change her tears into a big smile.

For the next couple of weeks I had radiation every day, which I did not enjoy. The only good thing about it was that I had made friends with one of the radiation students. I saw her every time I got my book signed. I was so happy when it was all over, I even drew a pretty picture to celebrate.

Miracles do happen

One day Mommy got a phone call from Dr Janine. She said that a famous Afrikaans singer who had very long hair wanted to get it made into a wig for a child who had no hair. Dr Janine wanted to know if I was interested, they were looking for a child who was well enough to meet her. I did not like wigs and thought I would look ridiculous in one. A few days later we went to meet her. Her hair was so long she could almost tuck it into her jeans. The TV cameras were there and so were the people from a magazine. They asked Mommy lots of questions about my cancer and my treatment.

A few days later we had to go to the wig shop where I was fitted with the wig. It looked pretty on me, but it was very itchy. A few days later we bought the magazine, which had my story and a photo in it. My story was also on TV, so I phoned all my friends and told them to watch.

Soon it was time for our suburb, Alberton's 100th Birthday party. Mommy's friends wanted me to go and meet the Mayor. There was a big party and I had to sit next to him. There were also a few famous people there who I met: Heinz Winckler, Amor, Vanessa Carreira and Mr Universe. They all wanted to know what was wrong with me. They took lots of photos with me and told me that I would be in the newspaper. My radiation burns were still very sore but I really enjoyed this outing.

At home we were digging a swimming pool, I could not wait for my treatment to be over so that I could swim. The garden was a mess and there had been a lot of rain, which meant a lot of mud.

At the end of the next month I had to start chemo again. The plaster that covered my Hickman Line was sticking to my skin and pulling it off was really sore. I could not help screaming and fighting. Then I had an idea, I told one of the nurses that if they left me alone, I would pull the plaster off myself. So they left me and told me to call them when I had finished. I took ages doing this and they got really irritated with me. They kept on coming in to see if I had finished picking it off. I had only managed to get one corner off, when one of the nurses told me that there were lots of other kids for them to sort out and that I must hurry up. There were many kids crying in the ward that day and I started crying softly, I wished I could be a normal kid and not have to do this.

Daddy was with me that day and told me to just pull the plaster off quickly and that it would be over. After a long time I got it off and the nurse came and cleaned out the Hickman line.

The next day was Mommy's birthday. Ben's mom popped her head into my ward and wished Mommy

"Happy birthday". She asked me how I was doing. The chemo was giving me terrible headaches and I felt as if my throat was closing and I could not breathe properly. My jaws ached. All the food tasted horrible, even my favourite bacon biscuits tasted yucky. Ben's mom explained that he had had the same kind of reaction to his chemo. I was glad when that chemo was over and that we were going home. I really wished that Ben was also well enough to go home. I loved my dogs and cats so much and always looked forward to seeing them.

The next week I had another checkup and a visit from Andrea. I never realized that she had helped me so much. I wasn't scared of finger pricks anymore. Andrea was happy with me. She wanted to see me the following week when I came in again for more blood tests. I really missed school and all my friends. They phoned me often and visited me when my blood counts were good.

I was keeping up well with my school work. Michelle would fetch the work from my teacher, I would do it at home and then she would hand it in for me. Mommy got notes from my teacher and helped me with my work.

I was booked in for another session of chemo between nineteenth and twenty-first of April. Ben was in hospital again. He was very, very ill and his mom was worried about him. His blood counts were extremely low and he had another infection. This block of chemo did not give me that horrible taste in my mouth. When the three days were over, I went home and ate well. A few days later Mommy got a phone call from Ben's mom who was crying hysterically on the phone. Mommy tried to calm her down and find out what had happened. Ben had passed away. We were all very, very sad. That was when we all realized how serious cancer is.

The next week I had another checkup. This time my blood count was very low (0.2) and I had to be careful not to get an infection. This blood count was supposed to be over 1. I had lost a lot of weight and now weighed 17kg. Mommy was keeping a close eye on me, checking my temperature often. I could see she was scared.

When I went for my next check-up it was the first day I did not fight to take off my plaster. I let Mommy do it without crying and screaming. My blood counts were up again, 1.4 so I was strong enough for my next dose of chemo.

The next week I was back in hospital for more chemo. My blood count was up to 5.2. The chemo was okay, this time I only vomited. We missed seeing Ben and his mom. I was tired of the hospital and got bored.

So I decided to sleep a lot.

Mommy and I used to pray together every night. We would always pray for me and for all the other kids in the ward. This time we said a special prayer for Ben's family. We also prayed for the doctors and nurses.

Mommy was very upset about Ben passing away. She was so scared that the same would happen to me. So we decided to ask God for a sign that I would be okay. Mommy told me that you have to be very specific with what you want from God, so that you could see that He had heard you and would answer your prayer. So she told God that she wanted to see a pink rosebud and that would be her sign that I would be okay. There were no flowers anywhere in the ward or in the garden outside. After our prayers I fell asleep. Nobody knew about our prayer and I wondered if God had heard us. The next day, when my chemo was over, we packed up our clothes and left the ward. Downstairs in the parking garage something strange happened. As we were walking to our car, Mommy stopped and stared. I asked her what was wrong. Stuck onto the side mirror of our car was a pink rosebud...

Moments In Time

A week later I was back for my weekly check-up. This time my blood count was a low 0.7. It was amazing to see how quickly the chemo knocked my blood count. I accidentally fell at home and my left knee was a bit sore. Mommy checked it and told me to rest it. She took me to see Dr Janine the next day because my knee had swollen up quite badly and I could not walk. It was very sore especially when Dr Janine pressed on it. She told Mommy to strap my knee with a bandage and told me not to walk on it. I had to use my crutches again.

On the twenty-second of May 2004 I was invited to the Miss Alberton finals. I was looking forward to it, but my temperature was 37.8°C and I did not feel well. Mommy and Daddy decided that I should not go to the finals and should rather stay at home with Granny. So Mommy, Daddy and Michelle went. They did not stay to the end because Granny phoned Mommy to say that she was worried about me because my temperature was climbing. They rushed home and Mommy checked my temperature, it was 38.2°C. She gave me two spoonsful of Panado. Later she took my temperature again, it had gone up to 38.4°C. Mommy was worried because the

Oncologists had told her to bring me into hospital if my temperature went over 38°C. So in the middle of the night she rushed me to Casualty at the Joburg Gen.

Two doctors checked me and I cried a lot because I was not feeling well and was tired. My throat was very sore. One of the doctors phoned the Oncologist who said I had to be booked in. All I wanted was to go back home. They wheeled me up to the ward and put me on a drip with antibiotics. I screamed and the nurses were cross with me for waking up the other patients - again.

The next day Dr Janine came to see me. She told Mommy that I would be in hospital for a minimum of five days. I was really upset because I was hoping she would give me some tablets and tell me to go home. She also checked my knee, which was still painful.

Soon I was feeling a lot better and was allowed to go home.

I hated walking with my crutches because they gave me blisters on my hands. I put a pair of gloves on which helped a bit but it was quite difficult because my hands slipped on the crutches.

Three days later I was back in for more chemo. I was happy for the break from using crutches, my hands were so sore.

My sister Michelle's birthday was on the second of June. She turned thirteen and she was going to have an ice-skating party that Saturday. I could not walk properly and was still struggling on crutches. I went with and watched everybody skate. I really wished I could skate too and asked Mommy if I could skate with my crutches. She laughed and said I was being silly. My aunt sat with me and kept me company while we watched everyone skate round and round.

A week later I went back to the hospital for another checkup. My blood counts were good. This time I met a new friend. Her name was Christy, she was a few months older than me. She had a brain tumour but it was not cancerous. She had just had two very long operations to remove the tumour. Her mom explained that she could not talk or move. I held her hand and spoke to her until she was tired. They had to feed her through a tube in her nose. Only her left hand worked, so she would squeeze my hand when I spoke to her. That is when I realized how lucky I was, even with my bad leg and sore knee. I spent a long time talking to her. Mommy made friends with her mom, so hospital life became a lot less boring.

Dr Janine came to check on me and asked Mommy if she would let me be on the **Moments in Time** calendar for the next year. The calendar would have pictures of people from all over the country who had cancer. Mommy agreed and set up an interview because they wanted to meet me first. Daddy took me to their offices and I met all the people involved with the **Moments in Time** project. Uncle Matt was the man who had started the project. We got along very well and he spoke to me for ages about my cancer and its treatment. He explained that all the money they got from the calendars and diaries would go to people who could not afford their cancer treatment.

Then the day came when they wanted to take photos of me for the calendar. They gave me a very pretty long pink dress with lots of shiny sequins on the front. Mommy took me to the change rooms and helped me put it on. It was too big for me, but they had explained that they wanted me to look as if I was playing dress-up with my mom's clothes. When I came out of the change rooms the lady who did the make-up, Ronel, helped cover up my Hickman Line with a big rose. Then she sat me on a chair and put a long blonde wig on me. Mommy said that the colour of the wig was very close to my natural colour. Then she put lots of makeup on my face. She even stuck little sparkles under my eyes and gave me a mirror and asked me what I thought. I looked so pretty. Then she called Michelle and put some make-up on her. She also looked beautiful. Next she gave me a pair of high-heels to put on. They were also too big for me and I could not stand in them without wobbling a lot. She told me I could put them on later just before they started taking photos of me. Then she adjusted my wig and put a crown on my head. The rose had moved and my Hickman Line was showing again so she fixed it.

Another lady came and told me how pretty I looked. My leg was getting sore from standing and I really wanted to sit down. Mommy was chatting to Ronel. Then the photographer, Jeanne-Claire called me. She wanted me to pose in front of the cameras. I had to put the high heels on and stand with my hand on my hip. Just as they were about to take the photo, my leg got weak and I called Mommy. She explained to Jeanne-Claire that my leg was very sore. She told me to sit down and rest a bit. Everybody was very friendly and told me how beautiful I looked. After a few minutes I got up and posed again. Jeanne-Claire took lots of photos and then they called Michelle and took some more of us together. When she had finished taking photos, they interviewed me. After that they interviewed Mommy, then Daddy and then Michelle. They explained that over the next few days they would look at all the photos they had taken and choose the best photos for the calendar.

Spunky

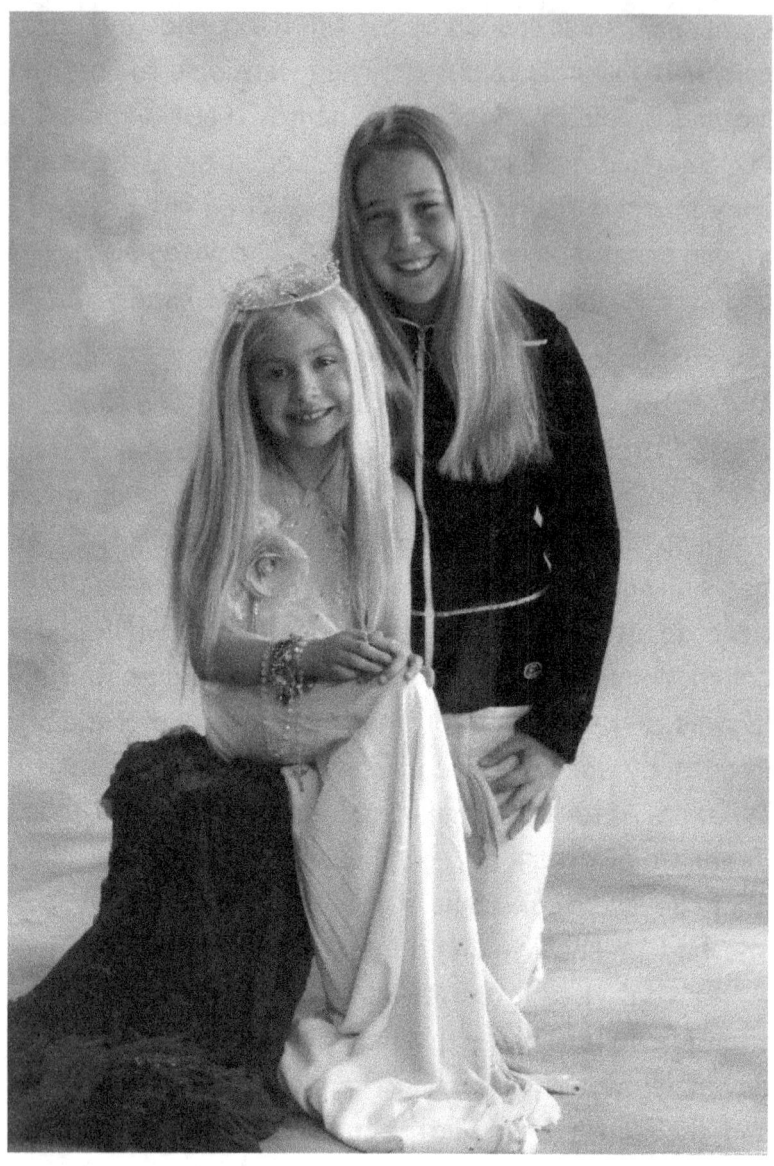

Me with Michelle at the photo shoot for Moments in Time

A week later I was back in hospital for my normal three days of chemo. This time it was fun because I got to spend more time with Christy. She was doing so well and was starting to talk again. My visits with her were quite short because the chemo made me feel sick and I vomited a lot.

Then something really sad happened. The little boy in the ward next door passed away. His family was very upset and there was a lot of crying and screaming coming from his room, so we went to Christy's ward where it was quieter. Mommy was very sad at this boy's death because she had been friendly with his mom. He had a kind of cancer that was very similar to mine.

At the end of that month I went back to the hospital again. My blood counts were good and my knee was getting better.

The following week Daddy took me for my check-up and my blood counts were excellent. I went to visit Christy but the nurse told us that she had gone home. I was so happy for her, she had been in hospital for about two months. At last I was finally off my crutches. It felt strange to walk without them, so I used just one crutch until I felt more stable.

I was looking forward to the eighth July 2004 - a while ago Mommy had spoken to a lady who wanted me to be in a TV advert. First, they wanted Mommy to e-mail a photo of me, which they had used on a Yoghurt leaflet. Then I had to meet them really early in the morning to film the advert. All the TV cameras were already there waiting for us. We spent the next eleven hours making the advert. We had lots of breaks in between and they gave us really yummy food. There were eight children in the advert altogether. I could not wait to see the advert on TV and told all my friends about it.

Two days later I was invited to meet Mr. Universe in Alberton City. They took some photos of me with him and the winners in all the categories of the **Miss and Master Alberton** finals. He was huge and I looked so small next to him. His leg was the size of my waist. I battled to get onto his lap. He was very friendly and chatted to me. Afterwards we had lunch with him at a pizza restaurant. Mr. Universe gave me a signed poster of himself.

Then I started chemo block number ten. I only had three more to go once this one was finished. I could not wait for it all to be over. While I was having my chemo, Mommy met a five-year-old boy in the ward, who also had Ewing's Sarcoma. His cancer spread to his thighbone and his lungs and they thought he was going to die. But he was completely clear and only came in for check-ups every three months. I was so happy to hear this.

I had another check-up and they said my blood counts were very low (0,7). I was not allowed visitors again and I had to stay at home. I was so bored and drew so many pictures, some were of the famous people I had met.

A few days later I went back to the hospital with Daddy. My blood counts were better (1,7). I was happy to see one of the CHOC volunteers. She was busy beading with some of the kids and told me to join in. I was glad because I was starting to get tired of all the hospital visits.

At my next check-up, my counts were an excellent (6,2). So I could have my third last lot of chemo. I vomited a lot and I just kept wishing that it was over, and that I could be at home. Then I got a surprise visitor. Christy came to visit me. She was talking and laughing. Her right arm had improved so much, it is almost like her left one. She was still going for physiotherapy to strengthen her body. She could also walk but only small distances. She said she might go back to school in September and was so happy.

I still got shocking pains in my leg. After the finger prick with Sr. Belinda, I fell outside her room. Sometimes my leg was not very strong.

Mommy took me for my next checkup, everything was fine. My knee was still very wobbly. Dr Janine phoned the physio who came to check my knee. They decided that I needed a knee brace to keep my knee stable. I had to bandage up my knee until I got a knee brace. The bandage helped a lot and I did not fall anymore. I then stopped waking up at night crying with pain. I went to see a doctor who made a knee brace for me.

Lion hug

Mommy and I were invited to the Alberton Civic Centre for a ladies' tea party for Alberton's Centenary Event on fourteenth August. We had to go on stage and I gave a talk about my cancer. Mommy was quite nervous, she hated giving speeches. Just before we went on stage, everybody was asked to enter a competition. Our speeches went well and afterwards everybody was crying and clapped a lot. A little while later they announced the winner of the competition. It was me. I had won first prize.

I was so excited and then they told me what I had won... R1000 worth of laser hair removal! Everybody laughed at me because I had no hair (not even one eyelash or eyebrow!) I also laughed. They said that I needed hair and did not need to get rid of it.

After another check-up at the hospital I had my knee brace fitted. It was very tight but the doctor said it would get looser with time. The physio also came to check on my knee. My blood counts were good (6,4) and when I had finished Mommy says she had a surprise for me. We were going away for the weekend. Her friend had invited us to a Lion Farm and she promised me that I would get to hold a lion cub. I loved lions and was so excited.

We stayed in a chalet and went on lots of game drives. It was so much fun. We saw impala, wildebeest, waterbuck, hippos, rhino's, and a fish eagle. We also went to a next-door farm where there were fifty-eight lions. They were all hand reared and we were allowed to touch them. The one cub was only a month old and I was allowed to hold him. A photographer was there taking lots of photos of us. There were two other cubs that were three months old, they played like kittens – biting our shoelaces and the bottoms of our jeans.

We went into a camp that had twelve cubs, they were bigger and we had to make sure that the cubs did not walk behind us, because they would bite our bums. We all really enjoyed that weekend.

I only had two more blocks of chemo left. We were all looking forward to the end of my treatment. Then Dr Janine gave me some good news… she said that I could go back to school when it was all over. This was the news I had been waiting for. I was not allowed to have any measles injections for two years after my treatment was finished. I also had to be very careful not to come in contact with anybody who had chickenpox, measles or mumps. If I did, I would have to tell the Oncologists straight away.

Lion hug

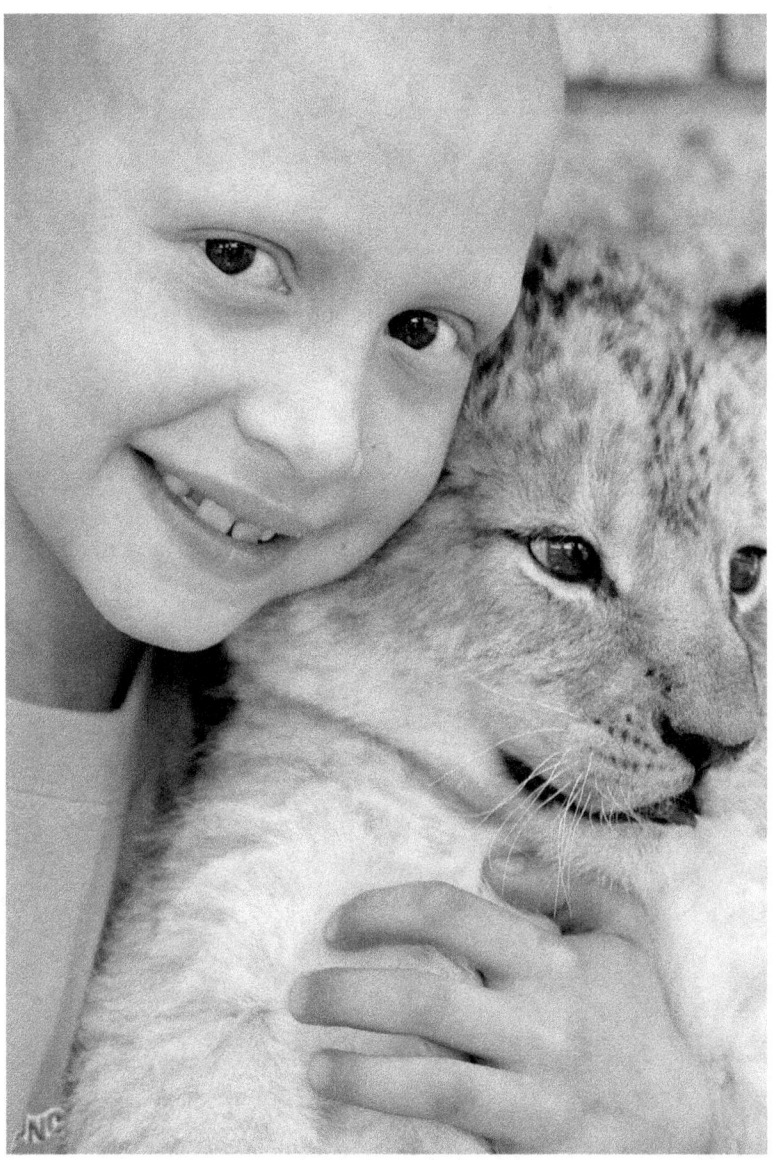

Me with Lion Cub

Spunky

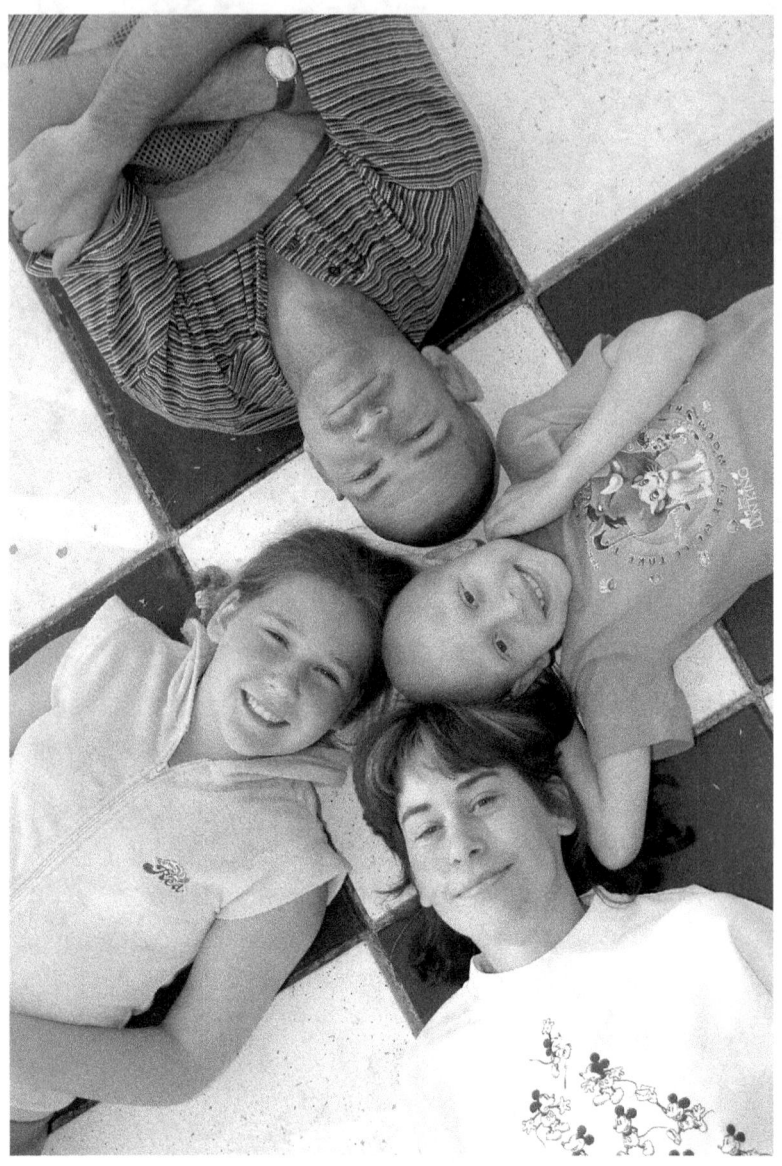

My family

Lion hug

Later that month I was invited to Sandton City for a CHOC Cow Parade. Daddy took me because Mommy had to go to work. We were met by Vanessa Carreira. She gave me a T-shirt and some paint. Then she showed me which cow I had to paint. There were lots of cows and lots of kids. It took quite a long time and we had a lot of fun. At the end the cows were auctioned off. I met some famous singers there, who autographed my T-shirt. My favourite was Danny K who chatted to me for a long time. My friend, Christy was also there, we had so much fun together. Every time I saw her she was getting stronger and stronger.

The next week I went for another check up. My counts were fine (2,9). After my check-up, my mom's friend took me to meet François Pienaar, a famous rugby (Springbok) captain. He was very big and very tall but very kind. I had often seen him on TV, it was nice to meet him. He picked me up and asked me how I was. I told him that I only had two blocks of chemo left. We met some other cancer kids and had to pose for a photograph where Dischem (a drug store) handed a cheque over to CHOC. After that I went to the recording studios for a TV interview. I was getting used to telling people about my treatment.

Spunky

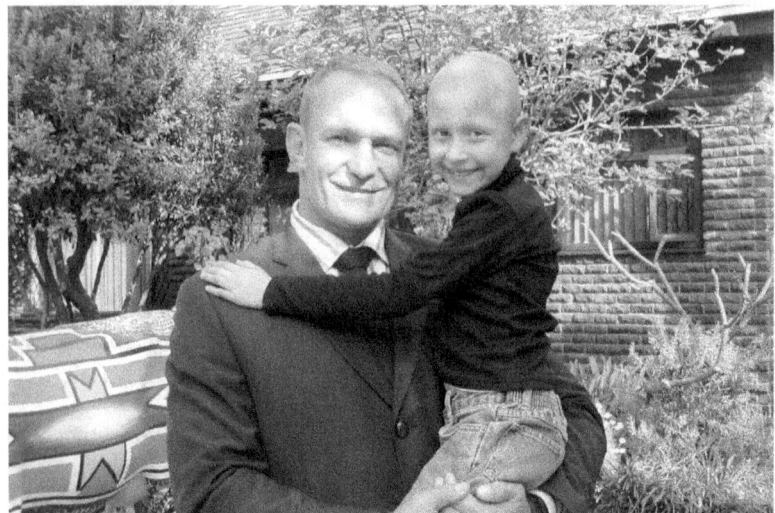

Me with Francois Pienaar

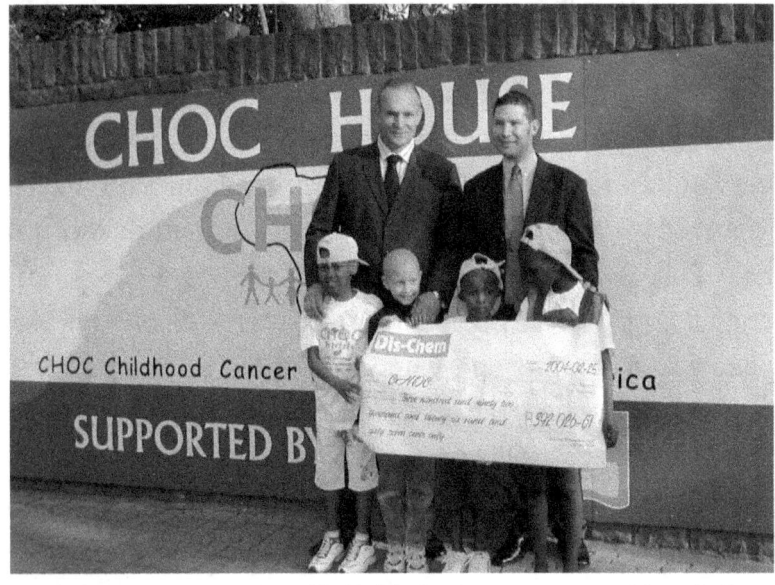

Handing over cheque to CHOC (Bottom row second from left)

Lion hug

When I next went into hospital for a checkup, the nurses were happy that I could take my plaster off quicker but I still cried because it hurt when they cleaned my Hickman Line. My checkup went well and my counts were fine.

In the middle of September 2004 I had my last block of chemo. I was so excited and hoped it would go quickly. I vomited a lot but I was used to that. Christy came to visit me. She could walk slowly now. She only came to the hospital for physio and speech therapy. She was doing so well.

Dr Janine came into my ward and told me that my Hickman Line must stay in for another six weeks. Then she gave me the good news. I was allowed to go back to school for the next term. YIPPEE!! I could not believe that some kids hated school, I had really missed it. Then she gave me some more good news. I could eat flavoured yoghurt again. She smiled because she knew that I had been waiting for that moment.

Mommy and I watched the last few drops of chemo drip into my arm. We cheered and clapped. Then the nurse came in and wanted to switch off my drip. I told her that I wanted to do it myself. She laughed and watched me while I flicked the switch with a big smile. One of my mom's friends came into the ward and gave me a big cup of yoghurt. She knew that I had been waiting for the doctor's good news. I knew that the other kids in the ward were not allowed to eat yoghurt, so I could not eat it in front of them. I rushed Mommy to pack up our clothes. All I wanted to do was get out of there and eat my yoghurt. As soon as we got to the car, I asked Mommy for a spoon. I gulped it down and finished it before we had even left the car park. It was so yummy. All the way home I was so excited and happy that all my blocks of chemo were over.

A week later Mommy got a phone call from Sr Susan. She asked Mommy if I was interested in doing another TV advert. This time is was an advert for the CHOC Childhood Cancer Foundation. A few days later two ladies came to visit us at home. They discussed the advert with Mommy.

Daddy took me to a house for the filming of the advert. It was a lot of fun. I had to bring some of my toys and dolls to make it look as if it was filmed in my bedroom. The producer of the advert explained to me what they wanted me to do. I sat at a desk and pretended to write a letter to my granny. My granny was supposed to be having her eightieth birthday and because I had cancer, I was scared that I would die before she would. I had to do it over a few times so that they had a few different ones to choose from. After that we had to go to a recording studio for a voice over. Here I had to record the words over and over and then they matched my voice to the actions in the advert. It was very interesting and they said I was really good at it.

I was not scared for my next check-up. My cousin took me to the hospital, my counts were good (1,6) and all the doctors were happy.

Great news

The next week I had another checkup. Some bad news... my blood counts were down (1,0) so I was not allowed to go back to school the following week in case I got an infection. I was really looking forward to seeing my friends and teachers again. Then the doctor sent me for a chest X-ray. My lungs were clear and I went home.

On Michelle's last day of school for that term she was called into the office. She was given an envelope to give to Mommy and Daddy. When Mommy opened it she burst into tears. The school had raised a lot of money and given it to us.

That night I noticed that my eyebrows were starting to grow in places. I still did not have any eyelashes or hair on my head. It was very annoying to open the car window because all the dust would fly into my eyes. I could not wait for my hair to regrow and to be able to open the window and have some hair blowing in the wind.

It seemed as if everybody wanted to talk to me. Mommy had a phone call from a well known TV talk show host. She wanted to interview me and discuss my treatment and the **Moments in Time** calendar that

I would be featured on the following year. I went to the recording studios and met her. I was a little bit nervous but she was so much fun and I relaxed quickly. Again I phoned my friends and family and told them when I would be on TV.

One day I got a letter in the post box that was addressed to me. I was very excited because I did not get letters often. I ran inside and showed Mommy. It was an invitation to the launch of the **Moments in Time** calendar. It would be held in a fancy hotel in Sandton early in October. A few days later Mommy got a phone call from a lady who wanted me to say a speech at the launch. She explained that they wanted me to talk about my cancer. That weekend we went shopping for something to wear to the launch. It had to be smart because I would be talking in front of lots of people. We bought a pretty dress and some silvery sandals. Mommy asked me if I wanted to have the sandals built up, but I thought they would look ugly. A few days before the launch Mommy helped me with my speech. She nagged me to practise it but I knew what had happened to me.

Soon the big day arrived. When we got to the hotel, all the people that I had met when they had taken photos of me for the calendar were there. It was good

Great news

to see them again. In the foyer there were big pictures of everybody who had taken part in the calendar. We all walked around and looked at them. My picture was there, I was going to be on the month of April. Soon it was time for the evening to begin. The doors to the hall opened and everybody started walking in. The hall was huge and suddenly I got nervous. A lady came and told Daddy that we had to sit in the front of the hall. All the people who were going to be on the calendar sat there with their families. First a lady got up and spoke, then she called Uncle Matt. He gave a speech and explained everything about the project. He showed a slide show of the making of the project and each page of the new calendar. When he was finished, Uncle Matt called me up onto the stage. Before I got up, Mommy wished me good luck and squeezed my hand. I did not like walking without a built up shoe and climbed slowly up the stairs onto the stage. Uncle Matt gave me a huge hug and then handed me a microphone. He asked me a few questions and then told me to give my speech. I got a bit nervous because there were about 500 people watching me. When I had finished everybody clapped and made a big fuss of me, and told me how well I had spoken and how brave I was. We met some TV celebrities and even Miss South Africa. We all went back into the foyer where they

Spunky

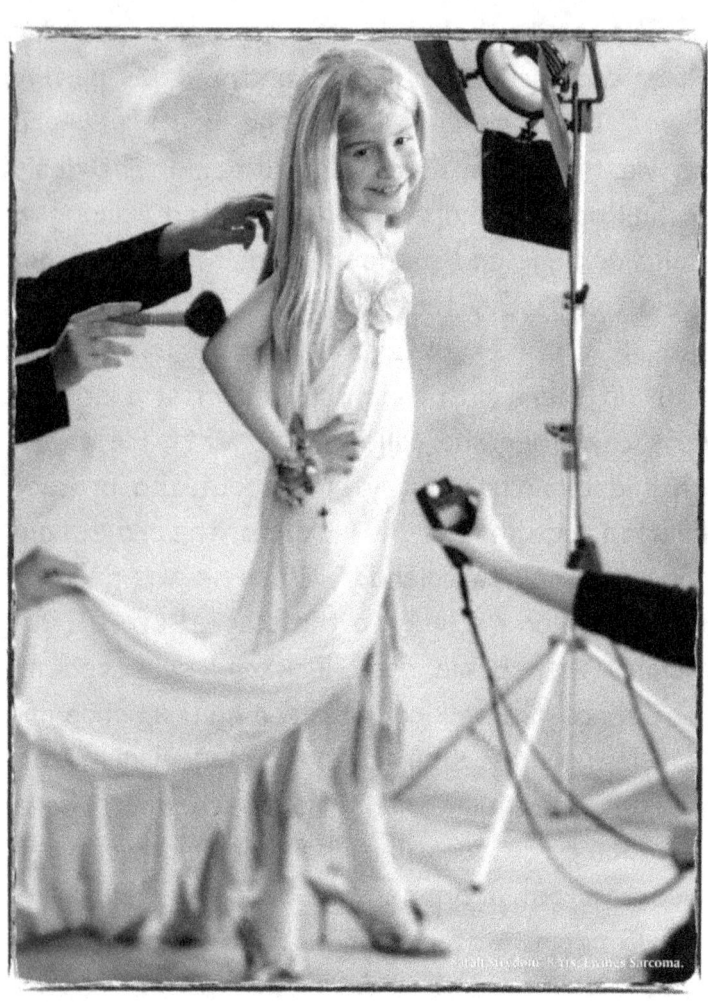

Moments in Time calendar April 2005
Photograph by Jeanne-Claire Bischoff

had lots of food for us. I did not get a chance to eat anything because everybody kept on talking to me. The launch finished late that night. I was so tired I fell asleep in the car on the way home.

Daddy took me for my next checkup. My counts were excellent (5,4) The next Friday I had to go to another hospital, the Donald Gordon, for an M.R.I. of my hip and leg. Dr Janine said that maybe after that, they would take my Hickman Line out. I was looking forward to that – then I would be able to lie down in the bath and swim again.

My eyebrows were starting to grow back. In some places they were about 1mm long. I only had two or three eyelashes regrowing. My head was still bald but well tanned because I played outside a lot. I watched Michelle swim everyday and wished I could jump in as well. I could also ride my scooter again because my leg was strong enough. I scootered around the house eight times – it was great fun. I wore my knee brace and limped a little bit when I walked. When I got tired my limp got worse. I was not using crutches anymore, sometimes when I battled, I used one crutch.

Uncle Andrew came to visit us again. I loved it when he visited us, we chatted for hours. He came with us on the fifteenth October 2004 when I had to go to the Donald Gordon Hospital for the M.R.I. of my hip and leg. This scan would show us if all the chemo and radiation had worked and killed off the cancer. The nurse had to use my Hickman line to inject the dye. I took my plaster off and screamed. It was very sore because my skin underneath was red and raw.

Uncle Andrew and Mommy waited with me while they did the scan. I couldn't hear them because this machine made a noise. When the scan was over we had to go to the Joburg Gen for a blood test and to flush my Hickman Line. My counts were excellent (6,7) and I weighed 19kg. I had also grown a little bit taller. Then we had to go back to the Donald Gordon Hospital to get the results of the M.R.I. We were all quite nervous. This was a big day for me. The nurse gave me the results of the M.R.I. in a big brown envelope. We drove back to the Joburg Gen without saying much to each other. As we walked into the waiting room at the Joburg Gen I saw one of my friends from the ward. She was just leaving and told me that her checkup went very well. Soon Dr Janine called us into her room. She asked me how I was and Mommy gave her the envelope. She read it carefully and then gave me the good news with a huge smile on her face. I was clear of cancer.

Great news

We were all very relieved and very, very happy. We hugged each other and started crying. It had been a very difficult time for us, but now it was over. Dr Janine explained that there was a lot of radiation damage inside my leg and a lot of scar tissue. Then she gave me some more good news. I was allowed to go back to school. I was SO excited. Mommy and I thanked Dr Janine for all her hard work and good treatment. Before we left she told us to make an appointment for my Hickman Line to be taken out. We had huge smiles on our faces as we walked out of the ward. Mommy phoned Daddy and gave him the good news. We phoned everybody we knew and shared our great news. That night we all went out for dinner to celebrate.

At last the day came when I could finally go back to school. I really enjoyed seeing all my friends and teachers again. Everybody crowded around me and wanted to know what had happened to me. I still had my Hickman line in and had to wear my knee brace, but I did not care, I was alive, and that is what counted the most.

Spunky

Let's celebrate

On the 20th October 2004 I was booked in for my Hickman line to be taken out. I was not allowed to eat or drink anything from ten p.m. the night before because they had to give me an anaesthetic. Mommy came into theatre with me. It was a quick procedure and they wheeled me out about twenty minutes later. When I woke up I was thirsty. This time Mommy knew to wait a while before she gave me something to drink. I was very hungry and asked her to get me some yoghurt. I just could not get enough of it and I was making up for all the months that I was not allowed to have any. She waited a while and later went to the shop and bought me some. After I had finished it, I vomited a lot, all over my bed. I had three stitches in my chest. I was very lucky that my Hickman line was kept clean because some kid's lines became infected. That was a big problem because they had to have them taken out before their chemo was finished.

The next week was my ninth birthday. A lot had happened to me in the last year. I was happy it was all over and just wanted to forget it all and live a happy normal life. I took cake and sweets to school for all my friends. That weekend I had a huge party at home.

Spunky

We celebrated my birthday and that I was clear of cancer. All my friends were there, they were so happy that I was well and back at school with them.

The following day Daddy took me to the hospital to get my stitches taken out. It was so good not to have any stitches or plasters on. I could not wait to go home and have my first proper bath for almost a year. At last I could lie down in the bath and not worry about getting the plaster wet. It was wonderful and I stayed in the bath for ages. Mommy even had to top up the hot water because it went cold.

Later that week it was very hot. Mommy said I could swim, because the holes from the stitches had closed nicely. I was a bit scared because I was not sure if I still knew how to swim. It had been a whole year. My leg was not strong but soon I was diving in and having great fun. It was so nice to swim with Michelle, instead of just watching her. The Oncologists had warned me that I must never allow my bad leg to be in the sun. I still had very bad radiation scarring which I covered with a long pair of shorts.

A few days later I was invited to the launch of the next **Moments in Time** calendar. It was held in the same hotel in Sandton. This time my best friend Roxy came along. We always had great fun together.

Let's celebrate

Uncle Matt, Ronel and all my friends from the calendar were there. I told them the great news that I was clear of cancer. Uncle Matt gave me a big hug and told me that he was so happy. Then we all started taking our seats in the big hall. The speeches began and Uncle Matt called me up on stage in front of about 700 people. He told everybody that I was clear of cancer and everybody started cheering and clapping. He asked me a few questions and then I went to sit next to Roxy again. When the speeches we over we all walked into the foyer. Everybody crowded me again and spoke to me for ages. The TV talk show host that I knew was there. She had tears in her eyes when she hugged me. The food was delicious and we all enjoyed the evening.

The following month I was invited to the CHOC Christmas Party held at the Joburg Gen. It was great fun, we all sang and danced. I saw a lot of my cancer friends from the hospital and all the Oncologists were there. They were happy to see that I was doing well.

On the twenty-fifth November, Michelle and I were invited to the Honours Evening at my school. I did not know what we were going to get and was really excited. Half way through the evening my headmaster called me up on stage. I had my knee brace on and was very careful when I walked up the

Spunky

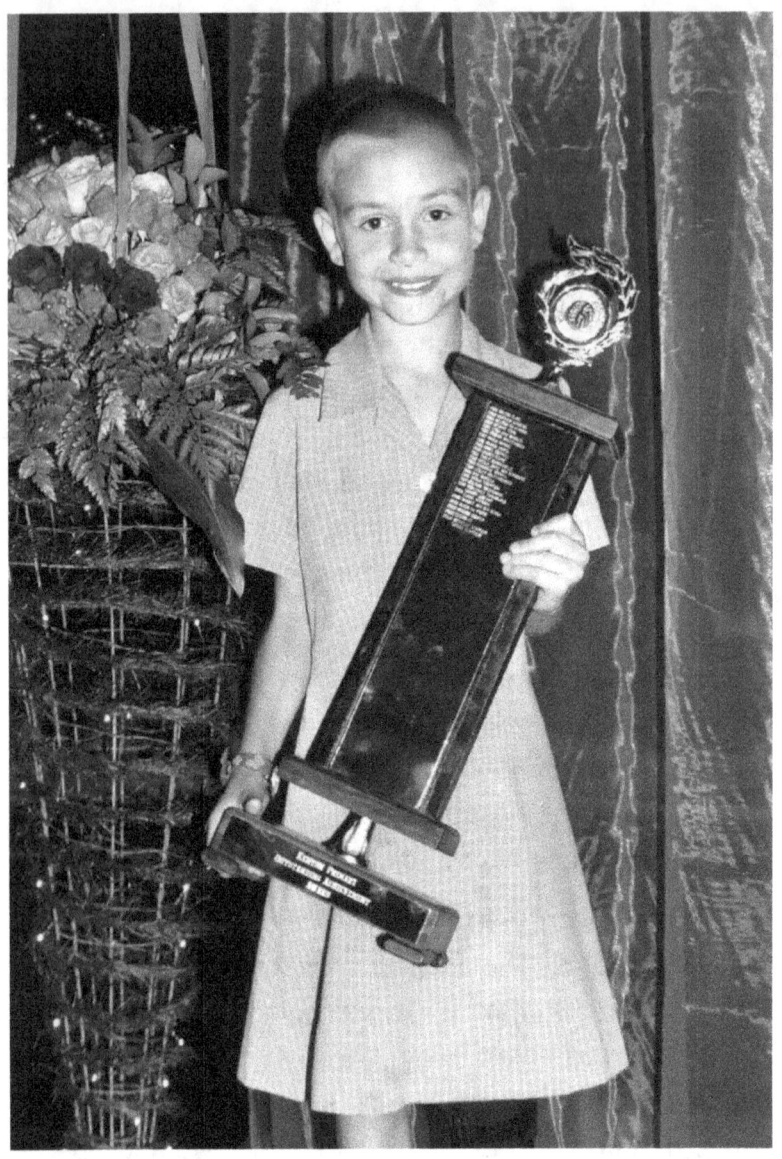

My Award for Outstanding Achievement

stairs. He explained my story to everybody and said that although I had been home schooled and had not been at school for three terms, I would be promoted to Grade four. Then he handed me a huge trophy for Outstanding Achievement. It was so big I could not carry it and one of the teachers helped me. Everybody in the audience got up and clapped for me. After that, Michelle was called up on stage and got an award for coping under difficult circumstances. Outside the school hall everybody wanted to talk to me.

Early in December Mommy took me to the Joburg Gen for a check-up. My blood counts were excellent (5,7). Dr Lee, one of the Oncologists, checked me and was very happy. My hair was growing nicely, it had also changed colour. Now it was darker than it used to be and a lot thicker. I looked as if I had a short haircut. She told me that I only had to go to the hospital for six weekly check-ups. Yippee.

We received a phone call from the producer of the CHOC TV advert that I had been in. She said that my advert had been entered in a competition and had come within the first ten in South Africa, and within the first three in the Best Concept category. The advert would definitely be shown on DSTV throughout 2005. We were given a copy of the advert on a DVD.

Not out of the woods yet

On the nineteenth March 2005 my dad's cousin invited our family to their house for dinner and so we went together in my uncle's Kombi (panel van). I had a lovely time playing with my cousins. We had just finished supper and were ready to go home. I was wearing my knee brace and we were playing a game. We were running down the passage to a bed and seeing who was the fastest, when I tripped over someone's legs. I screamed in pain as I collapsed on the floor. Everybody quickly ran upstairs to see what was wrong. I could not move my bad leg and Mommy picked me up and carried me to the nearest bed. Mommy and my aunt decided that I must go to hospital because something serious was wrong. They carried me to the Kombi and laid me on the back seat. While we were driving to the hospital, I felt every bump in the road and cried in pain.

Everybody was discussing which hospital to take me to but decided on the Johannesburg Gen because I was a cancer patient there and they knew my history. So they dropped Mommy and I off at 9:30.p.m and everybody else went home. As Mommy carried me into Casualty, I started vomiting. Mommy had to hold me over a dustbin, because there was nowhere else to vomit. Then she put me on a bed and I just screamed and screamed in pain. I had never been so sore in my whole life. We waited a long time and Mommy got angry with the nurses because they were not doing anything to help me. They weren't busy and were all chatting together. After a long time, a nurse came in and gave me a painkiller. I was shaking and very sore. Mommy wanted to phone Daddy to let him know what was happening but her cellphone's battery was flat. She didn't want to leave me alone there and asked the nurses to phone the Oncologists to let them know that I was in Casualty. They said they had but the next morning we found out that they had not. At about 2:30a.m., I was sent for X-rays. The radiographer was very unfriendly and told Mommy to straighten my leg. Mommy got angrier and told her that my leg was obviously broken and that I could not move it.

The radiographer said that she wouldn't be able to take the X-rays. She got angry and forced me to bend my leg. It was so sore, I could not stop crying.

Then I needed to vomit. Mommy told the radiographer and asked her for something for me to vomit in. She said she had nothing, and could not help us. Mommy found an old plastic container in the corner of the room, which I used to vomit in.

Not out of the woods yet

I didn't have anything to wipe my mouth with, so Mommy gave me the corner of the sheet on the bed to use. Mommy was shown the X-rays, which showed that my leg was badly broken, just below my hip joint. The break looked like a lightning bolt and there were small bits of bone around the break.

I was sent back to casualty and was given some more painkiller syrup. At about 5:30a.m. I was taken to the Orthopaedic ward. That ward was full of children in beds and their mothers sleeping on the floor next to them. Five nurses came in, and moved me onto a bed and started putting me in traction. First the nurses stuck wide Elastoplast all the way down my leg, then they connected that to ropes above my bed and then to water bags hanging off the end of my bed. I was in a lot of pain and screamed, "Mommy, Mommy, please just rather kill me."

Mommy was very tired, she had not slept at all and was crying. In between Mommy's tears, she told me that as soon as Daddy got there, we would go to a private hospital closer to home where we would get better treatment.

Daddy came at about 7:00a.m. and after that the doctor came in. He told Mommy, that he would re-assess me again on Tuesday morning as it was a long weekend.

He also said that I had to be in traction for the next eight weeks. Daddy was very angry and phoned for a private ambulance to get me out of there.

The paramedics arrived and they had a fight with the doctor who would not give them any information about me. Soon the paramedics came and took off the traction. Then they moved me gently onto a stretcher.

The one paramedic found that the machine that measures the amount of oxygen in my body wasn't working properly. It showed a reading of 52% and he said with that reading, I should have been dead. In the ambulance, they used their machine, which showed a reading of 94%. He was very cross and said that I had gone into shock and needed an emergency operation to fix my leg. Mommy rode in the ambulance with me. Daddy drove his car behind the ambulance. I do not remember much after that, because I was on a drip with morphine and felt very sleepy. I was being transferred to a hospital that was much closer to home.

When we got there a surgeon was waiting for me. He was very kind and took me straight into theatre. The anaesthetist came and gave me an injection. I couldn't really feel it and was still very sleepy. Mommy and Daddy were told to wait outside the theatre. After a long time I was wheeled out. The surgeon spoke to Mommy and Daddy. He had put a 10cm plate in my leg, which held my broken bone together. He said it was very badly broken and that he would see me later that afternoon. I was wheeled out of the theatre and into the Children's ward. When I woke up Mommy and Daddy were next to me. They were chatting to the nurses. The one nurse explained that Mommy could sleep next to me. She did not have a bed, but she could sleep on the couch at the bottom of my bed.

After a while the surgeon came to see me. He checked on the cut on my leg. He seemed to be happy and explained that I would be in hospital for the next eight days. The next day Michelle came to visit me. She slept next to me that night on the couch. She played a lot of games with me, it was so much fun. I was still on a drip and very glad to be free of pain. The nurses were fun too. They made the best two-minute noodles. I had many visitors while I was there.

Soon I was back at school. Mommy borrowed the little red wheelchair from the hospital. Every morning Mommy would meet my teacher. She would call one of the Grade seven boys to help me upstairs. Mommy carried me, my teacher carried my wheelchair and the boy had to carry my bag. I stayed upstairs all day and in the afternoon I had to be helped downstairs again.

Spunky

At home every day I would walk with crutches. I really wanted to go to school without the wheelchair. My friends were getting cross that I could not go onto the field with them. So at break I stayed in the classroom alone. I would often watch them out the window. They did not know how lucky they were, they could walk and run without any problems. They often complained about school and the teachers. I was just so happy to be back again.

At last, I went to school on crutches. Mommy still carried me upstairs because I was really slow getting upstairs on crutches. I got tired when I walked too far and my hands had blisters again. Soon I was able to walk quicker and get upstairs on my own. I hated going downstairs on crutches, it felt as if I was going to fall down the stairs. My teacher knew that sometimes I would be a little bit late for class.

One day after struggling upstairs I reached my classroom door. A big boy in my class was standing in the way. When I asked him to please move out of the way, he stayed there. I was really battling and just needed to sit down. My leg was very sore. He refused to move and started teasing me. He asked me if I got cancer on purpose to get attention. I was really cross with him. Eventually he moved out of the way.

For the next few days he continued to tease me. Other people were also asking me when I would walk properly again. One day I couldn't take it anymore and told Mommy and Daddy about it. They had a long chat to me and told me that nobody knew everything I had gone through and did not understand. They said that there would always be people teasing me and that I must try my best to ignore them. Then Daddy joked and told me to just whack them with my crutches. Some days I wish I could have.

A cheetah's touch

I was getting so used to doctor's check-ups. The Orthopaedic Surgeon said that the radiation had slowed my bone down from regrowing. He said that I must just give it time to regrow. I went for another cancer checkup. I had put on weight and now weighed twenty-two kg's. I had also grown a bit taller and was 124cm. My blood counts were still good.

At the next Orthopaedic Surgeon's check-up, he said that he was concerned about the difference in my leg length. He said that I might need to wear orthopaedic boots to make my bad leg the same length as the other one. He also told me that I must see another Orthopaedic Surgeon, Dr Richards who would be able to help me.

When I next went for a cancer checkup a few weeks later, I also had an appointment with Dr Richards. He told Mommy that an orthopaedic boot would put too much strain on my hip and leg (which was still broken). He measured the length of my legs and found that my left leg was twenty-five millimetres shorter than my right leg. He told Mommy to take me to an Orthopaedic Centre to get my shoes built up. He also said that the radiation had badly damaged my leg.

Two weeks later we went to the Orthopaedic Centre. They measured my legs again, to make sure that they would build up my shoes to the right height. They asked me to walk up and down the room a lot of times so they could see how I was walking. They put a heel wedge in my shoe to try and make my legs the same height. Then they made me walk up and down again. I was very tired when I got home from all that walking.

At the end of September, we were invited to the launch of the next **Moments in Time** calendar. This time I invited my favourite teacher. These launches were always sad because sometimes the people that featured on previous calendars had passed away. It was great to see Uncle Matt and my friends again. This time we met different TV celebrities. It was so nice to see them in real life. One of my friends from the hospital was there. He had leukaemia and had an infection. His mom and my mom were good friends and chatted for ages. They left early because my friend was not feeling well. I had been very lucky with my treatment, I had only had one infection during my chemo.

The next week I had another check-up at the Joburg Gen and the Orthopaedic Centre, which meant more walking up and down. They took the heel wedge out of my shoe and explained that it would be better if they built up my shoes instead. I gave them my school shoes to build up. Mommy wrote a letter to my teacher explaining that I would be wearing takkies for the next few days. Later that week we collected my shoes. The built-up heel really helped a lot. I was still walking with one crutch because my leg got really sore.

On the fifth November 2005 a lady from **Reach for a Dream** visited us at home. She was very friendly and talked to me for a long time. She asked me all about my cancer and how I was. Then she asked me what my three biggest dreams were. I was not sure what to say because there was a lot that I wanted.

She said "If you could have anything in the world, what would it be?"

I thought for a long time and then decided. My first dream was easy, I had always wanted to go to Disney World. I wanted to meet Mickey Mouse and all the other Disney characters. My second dream was to get a set of drums. I could already play the piano and wanted to start another instrument. My third dream was to get a PlayStation 2, all my friends had one and I also wanted one. The lady wrote down a lot of things and then told Mommy that they always tried their best to make a child's first dream come true, if they really couldn't then they would go on to the second dream.

She asked Mommy many questions and wanted to know if we had ever been overseas. We had never been outside South Africa. She spoke to Mommy for a long time about the costs involved. I could not believe what I was hearing that night I could not sleep and kept on wishing that my dream would come true.

Three days later I had to have more X-rays of my leg. The bone still hadn't healed.

Later that month I was invited to two Christmas parties, one at the Radiation Department in Hillbrow Hospital and the other one at the Joburg Gen for the cancer kids. I had a lot of fun seeing some of my old friends again.

Early in the New Year, I handed in a pair of takkies to be built up. My leg was still sore but the shoes helped me a lot. I had another check-up at the Joburg Gen and some chest X-rays. Everything was clear. In February, I had to go for a C.A.T. scan of my leg. I knew what they were going to do and did not fight with the nurses. The results were good, there were no cancer cells in my leg. We were all very happy because we were worried.

The next week I had another check-up at the Orthopaedic Centre. I was walking with a bad limp and they found that my back was skew when I walked, but straight when I sat down.

A cheetah's touch

At last some fun. I was invited by **Reach for a Dream** to go to a camp in Brits. There were many other kids there, all with life threatening diseases. I knew some of the kids from the cancer ward. It was great to see them again. We slept in Wendy houses (play houses) on bunk beds. It was fun from start to finish. We played many games and we learnt how to shoot with a bow and arrow. I battled a bit in the beginning, but was soon hitting the target. There was a kind man named Smiley, the camp leader, who was extremely funny and made us laugh, telling us jokes, acting out plays and dancing around, every morning before we prayed. Early one morning we went on a game drive. We saw many animals and enjoyed it. Later that day we were allowed to go to the elephant camp. We were all very excited when we climbed into the bakkie (utility car). We walked in between the elephants. I was so surprised at how big the elephants were. We all touched the elephants, played with their eyelashes and felt their feet. In a way, I was scared they would squash me, but I was so excited to see them to. They were so big and beautiful and we were allowed to feed them. Every group of two had a big trough, which included large bowls of green, stinky mashed grass, that we had to feed them with our hands. We also had some fruit, then the greatest part – we got to ride on them.

Spunky

Smiley helped me up onto the big elephant, and I felt on top of the world. My friend Kayla, who was also new to the camps, looked at me and giggled. I wished Mommy was there, because 'ellies' were her favourite animal and she would have been so happy to ride one. After walking around the big farm, we got off, went back to our 'camp home', and we played 'Seek the Lantern'. There were two teams, the hunters and the seekers. Kayla and I were on the same teams for everything, so we became seekers together. The hunters had to find us and catch us before we got to the lantern, which was hidden far away on the farm. Kayla and I were laughing so much, we rolled in mud so the hunters with big torches didn't spot us, but we could not hold in our laughs. We finally made it to the lantern, we shared the prize together, the biggest slab of chocolate we had ever seen.

That night we both slept at the top of our bunk beds, which were next to each other. We had to be quiet, because the camp leaders were outside talking. They would come in and tell us to go to sleep if they heard us. So, whispering, and trying to hold in our giggles, we pulled funny faces at each other. It was about midnight, and we were having so much fun, we did not want to go to sleep.

A cheetah's touch

The next day, Kayla and I snuck out early in the morning to look at the animals. We were not allowed to touch them. There was a big pig, it was a black and white bush pig. So we snuck into its pen and tickled it and touched it. Smiley caught us but didn't do anything as the next day we were going to touch it anyway. After that, he told us to meet him next to the swimming pool. We were going on an adventure.

I wore jeans and a t-shirt, which I didn't want to get dirty but Smiley shocked us when he said, "Today, we are having a Mud Obstacle Course" Kayla and I looked at each other, as we wore our best clothes, and didn't have time to change. So we crawled under nets, slid in mud, threw mud balls at each other, getting grass and mud in our hair. Smiley saved the best for last - a long wet muddy slide. Kayla and I did not care about our clothes, we sped down the slide and then jumped in the pool, making the water an ugly brown, but we did not care, because we were having the greatest fun ever.

The next day we went to a cheetah sanctuary and we were allowed to touch a teenage cheetah. He was so cute and had been touched by over 2 000 people. We were not allowed to touch his head because he would bite us. We also learned how to call each other using drums. In the mornings we had very yummy breakfasts. We also saw a small lizard and three snakes, which we could hold if we wanted to. I made lots of new friends there.

My hair had grown just over my collar. I had been trying for ages to make a pony tail but it wasn't long enough. Now at last I could do it. Mommy helped me to tie it up for school. I thought about all my friends probably did not even think about these things. I had to take more time off school for another checkup with Dr Richards. He looked at the X-rays and was worried. My leg was still broken after a whole year. No wonder it was still sore and I couldn't walk properly.

I had to go back a week later to see a panel of Orthopaedic surgeons at the Joburg Gen. As we walked into the room, there were about thirty doctors waiting for us. Dr Richards was there and explained to them what had happened to me. Then they all checked my leg and asked me to walk up and down the room. As soon as I stopped they asked me to walk again, and then again. They discussed my X-rays for a long time and eventually told Mommy that we must wait another two months to see if my broken leg would heal on its own. They said if it did not, then I would need an operation to force it to grow together.

Two weeks later I was invited to another **Reach**

for a Dream camp. This time it was held in Nelspruit. I loved these camps and was so excited. We all met at the Joburg Gen and left in a bus. On the way there we all chatted and cracked jokes. When we got to the camp we unpacked our bags. After lunch we went on a game drive. The weather was beautiful and we had a lot of fun. We stopped at a river and they taught us how to fish. I didn't catch any but one boy caught a big catfish. That night we had a braai (barbecue) and sang songs around the fire.

The next day everybody was excited. They told us that we were going on a plane ride. We all climbed into a small plane and flew over Nelspruit. We flew above the forests, it was so beautiful. When we landed, we all had something to drink and later we could go horse riding. I was really looking forward to it but all of a sudden I felt sick and started vomiting. One of the **Reach for a Dream** ladies told me to rather stay with all the camp leaders and not go horse riding. I was upset but she explained that I would feel worse if I went riding. That night we toasted marshmallows over the fire. The next day we all slept on the bus on the way home.

In the middle of May **Reach for a Dream** invited me to Rand Airport. We were taken for a ride in a helicopter. We flew over the middle of Joburg and then back again. It was great fun. I loved the way the helicopter landed, it was so cool. Then we went on an old Jumbo 747 which had been converted into a museum. My leg was very sore because I had fallen at school a few days before. I was back on crutches and was really battling. We were shown all over the Jumbo, I even got to sit in the pilot's seat. Daddy picked me up when we had left the plane.

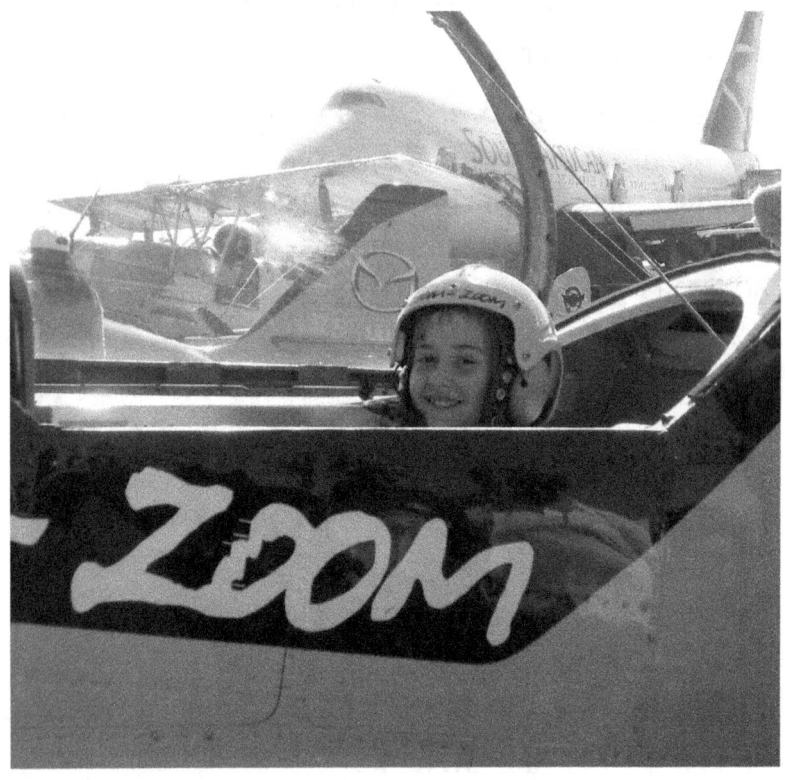

Me in a plane

A cheetah's touch

One of the men from Reach for Dream came and asked me if I wanted to have a ride in a small aeroplane. He carried me to the plane and made sure I was okay. Michelle was also allowed to come for the ride. I always felt sorry for her because often she felt left out. I loved flying over the highways and seeing all the tiny cars down below.

We flew out to Sandton City and there we met two small planes in the sky. They did all kinds of tricks over our plane. One of the pilots waved to us from his upside-down plane next to ours. Then I suddenly felt very sick. I told one of the ladies who had come with us. She gave me a cap to vomit into. I was glad that we were on our way back to the airport. When we landed there were a lot of planes practising for an air show that was on the next day. A TV crew had arrived and interviewed us. Photographers took photos for articles that would be in the newspaper the next day. I met more famous people. They spent a long time talking to us. We all were given T-shirts and I got everybody to sign mine. After this we were called into a hall and had a party.

Snap

In the middle of June that year Daddy took me to the hospital for X-rays. The next day I had to see Dr Richards. He had really bad news for us. The plate in my leg had snapped in half. He was quite shocked, because that was never supposed to happen. My leg was still broken. I had to have another operation to remove the broken plate. He explained that he was going to put in a 'blade plate', which was a plate attached to a blade that would go through my hip joint. I was not looking forward to this, it sounded so sore. He also said that he would take some bone from my hip to help my bone heal. Then he gave me some more bad news. I wasn't allowed to go back to school. I was also not allowed to walk at all and had to either use a wheelchair or two crutches. He said that if I tried to walk there was a good chance that my whole hip joint could collapse. I had to be very careful.

After this I went to the Joburg Gen for another checkup. Dr Lee, one of the Oncologists, was very sad to hear that I would need another operation. My throat had been a little bit sore and she told me that I had tonsillitis. She gave me antibiotics and told me that I had to be well otherwise they would not be able to operate on me.

On the twenty-third of June I had to be at the Flora Clinic very early in the morning. I was worried and so was Mommy. The operation went well and when I came out they put me in ICU with four premature babies. The first night I was there I was on morphine, so I slept very well but for the next three days the screaming babies irritated me. Mommy wasn't allowed to sleep in the ward with me and I missed her a lot. Soon I made friends with the nurses in ICU and then I was transferred to the Paediatric ward.

They put me in traction to keep my leg and hip straight. It was very uncomfortable and I could not turn over or move in my bed.

Mommy used to visit me very early in the morning, then go to work. At lunchtime she would pop in for a quick visit and go back to work. As soon as she finished work she came back and stayed with me until I was tired. I begged the nurses to let Mommy sleep in the ward with me but they wouldn't. I stayed in hospital for a week. This hospital was quite far away from home, so Mommy was glad when I was finally allowed to go home. When I got home, my friends and family came to visit. Mommy had borrowed the little red wheelchair again. After the holidays I went back to school and again my teacher and Mommy carried me upstairs. The kids in my class teased me and told me that I was acting and looking for attention. They didn't know how much I wanted to run around the field and run up the stairs.

Two weeks later my wound was getting red and Mommy took me back for a checkup. The Orthopaedic surgeon had a look and told me that an abscess had formed and he booked me back into hospital. I was very angry. I was back in hospital for the next four days on antibiotics. I cried a lot and wished I could be like everybody else.

Early in August **Reach for a Dream** invited me to a Rally Day, which was held at Gold Reef City. We were all supposed to run in a rally. My leg was still sore and we just waited for everybody to finish their run. One of the ladies from **Reach for a Dream** asked me if I would go up on stage in front of everybody to receive a cheque for **Reach for a Dream.** I went up on stage with PJ Powers, a famous singer and collect the cheque. The photographers were there and the next day I was in the newspaper again.

Two weeks later I was invited on to a TV game show. Only cancer children were invited because the theme of the show was cancer awareness. When we arrived at the studio we were shown into a room, which had been made into a basketball court. We were divided into teams and they explained how the ball games would be played. My leg was still weak, so I couldn't run properly but I had a lot of fun. I was very good at the games where I had to throw the ball. Some of my friends had watched it on TV and told me how lucky I was to be invited onto the show.

The next week I had an appointment with Dr Richards. My wound was healing well and he was happy with my progress.

Dreams do come true

Early in September 2006 Mommy got a surprise phone call at work. It was from the lady from **Reach for a Dream**. She told Mommy that all the arrangements had been made to make my first dream come true. We would be flying to America for a week and staying in a village called '**Give Kids the World**'.

Mommy fetched me from school that day and could not stop smiling. I climbed into the car and asked her why she was so happy. She looked at me and shouted, "We're going to Disney World."

I could not believe what she was saying. I think we were the noisiest people on earth that day, we were so excited. As soon as we got home we went on the Internet to see what Disney World and **Give Kids the World** was all about. That night I went to bed really late, everybody was talking about our first trip to America. I could not believe that my dream was coming true.

The next few weeks we were busy sorting out passports and visas. I had to apply for an unabridged birth certificate. We were going to fly to America on the ninth of November and come back a week later. It was very far to travel for just one week but I was so happy.

Then another miracle happened. Mommy was talking to one of her customers about our trip and he offered us his timeshare in Orlando. Now we would be going to America for two weeks.

I wished that time would go quickly until our holiday and then that it would slow down a lot while we were there. If only I had a time machine...

Before we left I had more check-ups with Dr Richards and the Oncologists. They heard all about our trip and wished us well.

Two days before we left, our visas still hadn't arrived. Daddy and Mommy were worried and did not know if we would be able to go to America or not.

Then we got a phone call we were all waiting for, to say that they were ready. We made a big list of all the things we needed to take. It was so exciting. Daddy asked his friend to look after our house and our pets while we were away. I hated leaving our animals behind.

Our flight was at 6:25p.m. on the second of November 2006 so Daddy's friend took us to the airport and told us to have a great holiday. We were all very excited. My leg was a lot better and I was only using one crutch now, it helped me to balance. Before we got on the plane we walked around the shops at the airport.

Then suddenly I slipped and fell. My knee was very sore. Mommy picked me up and carried me to the bathroom. I was crying a lot. I wished I had brought both my crutches along.

Daddy carried me onto the plane. I was really happy when I finally sat down. We all could not believe that we were actually going to America. I had never been on such a big plane, and wondered what we would get for supper. The air hostesses walked up and down, giving us whatever we wanted to drink. In front of our seats were small TV's and we could watch movies or play games. Michelle quickly found **The Pirates of the Caribbean** - she loved Johnny Depp. Soon it was time to eat. We had a choice of either beef stroganoff or chicken stew. I chose the beef, it was delicious. We watched more movies and then we were given a small plastic bag. In it was a fold-up toothbrush, the smallest tube of toothpaste I had ever seen, a face cloth, a pair of socks and a blindfold. I was sitting next to Mommy and we both joked about how funny we would all look wearing our socks and blindfolds. Mommy helped me to the bathroom. None of us could sleep on the plane, we were all too excited and wondered what America would be like.

The next morning we landed in Dulles International

Airport in Washington at 6a.m. As we got off the plane, we caught a shuttle, which drove us from where the plane landed to the airport. There were signs everywhere, so we knew exactly where to fetch our luggage from. Daddy checked our tickets for our next flight. The flights were booked from Baltimore Airport to Orlando at 4.45p.m. We did not even know where Baltimore was. So Daddy went to ask a lady behind a desk. She told us that we could catch a cab to Baltimore, it was not far from Washington. We went outside to where all the cabs were parked. It was freezing. We did not think it would be that cold.

Daddy found a cab driver who told us he would drop us off in the middle of Washington and come back for us later. Daddy asked him what we could do with our suitcases because we could not walk around with them. He told Daddy that he would keep them in his cab and bring them back later. He gave Daddy his phone number and said he would meet us that afternoon at 2.30p.m. When he left, Mommy laughed and said that she did not trust him and that he wouldn't be back and had left with all our belongings.

We walked across the road into a beautiful park with pretty flowers everywhere. There were many squirrels running up and down the trees. We found a little coffee shop in the middle of the park. We bought some really yummy hot chocolate to try and warm up. My leg was really sore, so Daddy carried me on his shoulders. We walked all around, looking in museums, art galleries and even walked up to the White House. The queue there was very long so we did not go in. On our way back we went into McDonald's for lunch. It was the biggest McDonald's I had ever seen. We were surprised to see that they sold salads there, at home they only sold burgers.

We all wished that we had brought warmer clothes, we were shivering and our jaws were aching because our teeth were chattering so much. Then we walked back to the place where we had to meet the cab driver. At exactly 2.30p.m. he arrived with our luggage. Daddy just smiled at Mommy. He was very friendly and helped us into his cab. He drove along a highway with the most beautiful trees. It was autumn and the leaves were all shades of red, gold, brown and yellow. Behind the trees we could see a very wide river. The cab driver chatted to us and asked us where we were from.

We arrived in Baltimore, paid the cab driver and thanked him for his help. He wished us well and told us to enjoy his country. Baltimore airport was smaller than Washington's. Before we climbed on the plane to fly to Orlando, we had to put our hand luggage through an X-ray machine. Then we were shown to a different section where they sprayed us. I asked Daddy what they were doing and he said they had to spray us because we came from Africa. I felt like a bug. Then a man came up to us and told us to walk through another X-ray machine. As I walked through this machine, a lady stepped forward and told me that I must go through it again without my metal crutch. She did not know how sore my leg and knee was. Mommy tried to help me through it but the lady said I had to walk through on my own. I was angry with her and battled. After that Daddy carried me onto the plane. We were very tired, irritated and very thirsty but there was nothing to drink on that plane.

We arrived in Orlando at 9.00p.m. and were met at the airport by a very friendly man and his wife, who came from **Give Kids the World**. They were holding up a board that said "Welcome Sarah Strydom." They chatted to us and asked us how our first day in America had been. We were exhausted and just wanted to sleep. They dropped us off at the timeshare and told us that they would see us in a week's time. They wished us a wonderful holiday and told us to contact them if we needed anything.

The timeshare was beautiful. We were staying upstairs, so Daddy carried me up. They did not have keys for the doors, we had to slip a card into the lock, which opened the doors. The beds were absolutely huge and I could not wait to fall asleep. We did not unpack our bags and all just fell asleep in our clothes.

The next morning the first thing we did was find a shop. There was one in the timeshare. We bought some food and cool drink. There were very big gardens, with lakes and fountains everywhere. After our breakfast we walked around. There was a huge swimming pool with palm trees and a big entertainment area for kids. We spent a lot of time there, just relaxing. The weather was beautiful, much warmer than in Washington.

That afternoon Daddy hired a car so that we could see what America was like. When it arrived he called us downstairs. In the parking lot was a beautiful white Pontiac, which Daddy had hired for three days. We took a ride to Wal-Mart, which was close by. Daddy was a good driver and quickly learnt how to ride on the other side of the road.

Walmart was amazing. It was the biggest shop I had ever seen. We spent the rest of the day walking around looking at all the things that we have never seen before. There was lots and lots of Disney stuff. Even the food aisle was interesting it had a huge selection with new flavours we had never heard of.

Spunky

When we got back to the timeshare, Michelle asked Mommy to play tennis with her. They caught a shuttle up to the courts and Daddy and I stayed behind. I played with my new Barbies and tried the new sweets and biscuits we had bought.

The next day we got up early because I wanted to see the entertainment area. It was a big arcade with lots and lots of games. Daddy and Mommy loved the car racing machine. We played a lot of shuffle board. Then we spent the rest of the day at the pool again. Michelle and I floated on the tubes around the palm trees. It was so beautiful. Mommy and Daddy lay on hammocks in the sun.

Every night Mommy and Michelle played their games of tennis. I really wanted to join in but my leg was still a bit sore. Mommy told me I should rest. I decided to fetch tennis balls for them instead. As I was fetching one, my leg just collapsed. I could not get up and started crying. Mommy ran over and picked me up. She took me to the reception area and then we caught the shuttle back to our unit. She carried me upstairs and laid me on my bed. My knee was very sore. Early the next morning Mommy and Daddy went to the nearest chemist to buy me some painkillers and some ointment to rub on my knee.

I rested on the couch with pillows under my knee. That afternoon we took a drive around Orlando. There were lots of shops everywhere selling Disney things. Mommy and Michelle investigated all the shops and sometimes when my knee was too sore, Daddy and I stayed in the car and waited for them.

Very soon the week was over and we had to leave. I was sad because I had really enjoyed resting and relaxing. My knee was a lot better now. We packed up our things and caught a cab to **Give Kids the World**. We had read on the Internet about this village, it looked so exciting.

Never let the fun end

As soon as we arrived we were met by a lady who welcomed us and showed us around. Everything in the village was just for kids. We walked out of the reception area to a magical castle, with a small knight standing at the wooden door as you crossed over the drawbridge. He greeted us as we walked past. As we entered the castle we could not believe our eyes. There was so much to do. There was a huge book and you could watch a screen and make up your own fairytale by pushing buttons on the book.

In another room there was a huge cupboard full of clothes that you could dress up in. You could be a queen in a velvet dress with a crown or a joker in a multi-coloured suit. There were all kinds of games to play and even a pillow machine, which made your very own pillow.

As we walked into another room in the castle, the lady showed us hundreds and hundreds of stars on the ceiling. Each child who had been to this village was given a mirror cut into the shape of a star. They had to write their name on it and the date and the stars were stuck up for everybody to see. She explained that later in the week, I would get mine.

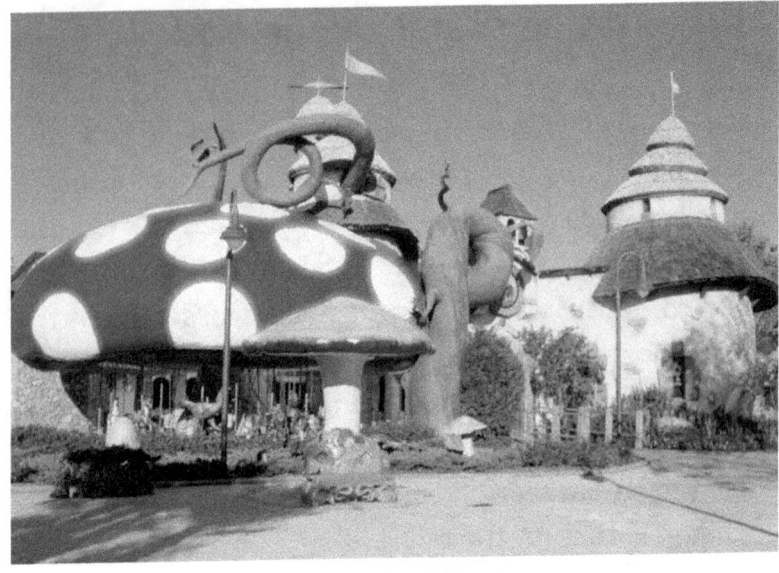

The Castle of Miracles

As we walked out of the castle I noticed that the paving bricks in the road had people's names on them. I asked her what they were for. She explained that you could buy a paving brick and the money would be donated to the village. We were so busy reading people's names that we did not see the dining room in front of us. It was in the shape of a Gingerbread House.

Inside were rows and rows of hundreds of different kinds of dolls from all over the world. The tables were brightly coloured with thousands of peppermints under the glass. We were told what time the meals were and that there were plenty of helpers who would serve us.

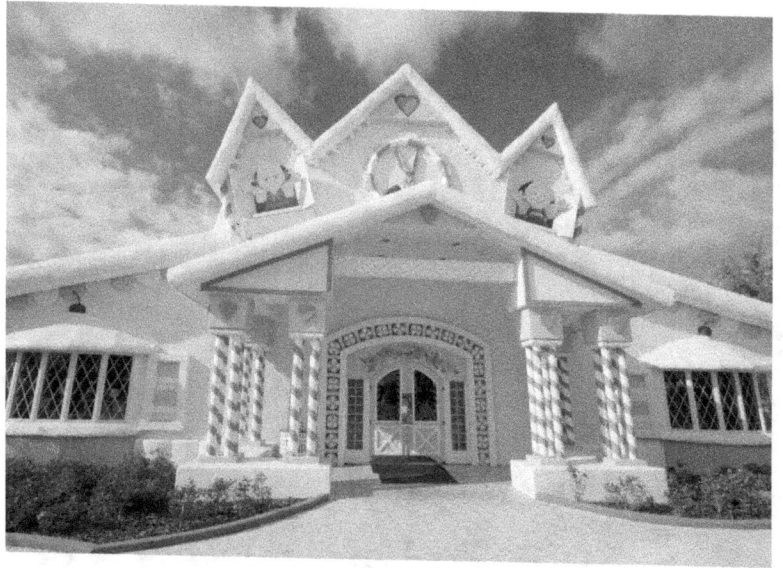

The Gingerbread House

Then we went outside and passed a huge carousel. There were brightly painted horses waiting for kids to ride on. The house we were staying in was just outside the Gingerbread House. As we walked past an old tree, it suddenly started snoring. We all looked at each other in surprise and burst out laughing. The lady explained that that was Ol' Elmer who had been snoring for years. In his trunk we could see his closed eyes and open mouth.

As we walked across the beautiful garden to our house, we saw that our name had been put on the signpost to show us that was where we stayed. Our house was cosy inside with everything we needed.

Spunky

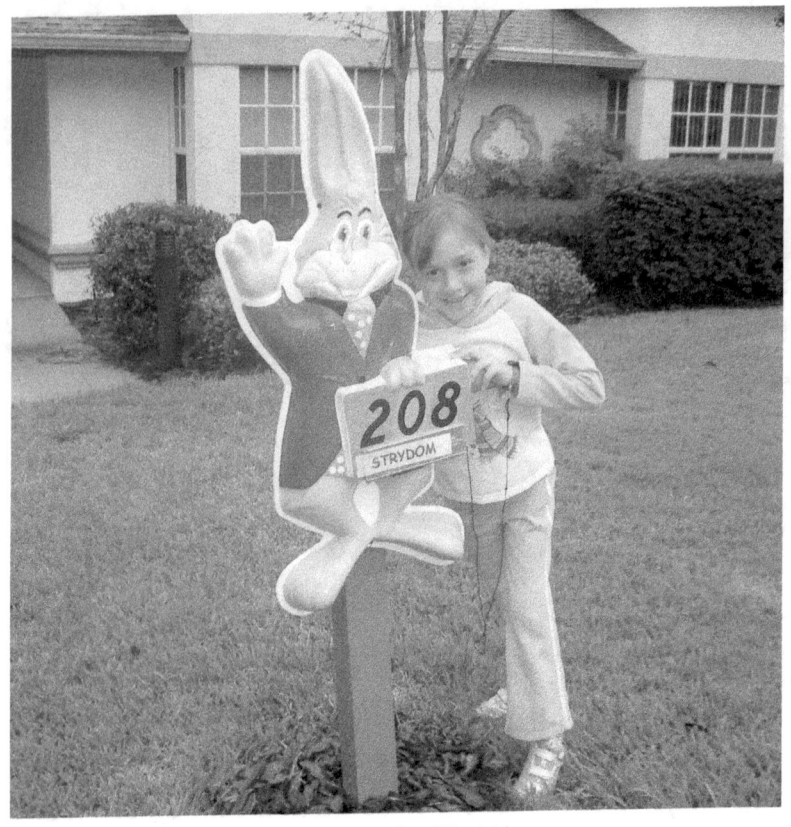

Our Give Kids the World house

Then the lady took us back outside and showed us a huge swimming pool. She explained that only children with life threatening diseases could visit this village. She said that kids from all over the world came here. On both sides of the swimming pool was a ramp for children in wheelchairs. At the other end there were lots of sprinklers to run through. There was a table and chairs underneath a roof that was held up by giant orange carrots. Next to it was a huge rabbit.

Then we walked into Julie's Safari Theatre. Here she explained that various Disney characters would be visiting throughout the week. She said we would be getting a programme to let us know what would be happening. She explained that everything in the village was free, we could even use the phone to call home if we wanted to.

Before the lady left us, she showed us an entertainment area. There was a table tennis table, darts, a huge TV and then my favourite game of all, driving remote control boats. We were the captain of a ship and had to steer the tiny boats outside on the water using big wooden steering wheels. As we walked out, I knew that this trip to America would be one I would never, ever forget. We went back to the reception area, collected our bags and went to our house. We unpacked our clothes into the huge cupboards and then walked around the village.

That evening we went to the Gingerbread House for supper. We were starving but not for long. We were welcomed and handed trays for our food and then told to help ourselves. The selection of food was huge.

Some of the food looked a bit strange and Mommy had to ask what it was. It was fun eating food that you do not get back home.

After supper we walked around the village and found the Ice-Cream Parlour. We could have any ice-cream we wanted. There were ladies behind the counter serving us and laughed when we battled to decide what to eat. The selection was too big. After choosing the flavour, the next problem was deciding what sauce and what topping to have on it. There were nuts, chocolate sprinkles, M&M's the list was endless. As we walked out the lady behind the counter reminded us that we could come back as many times as we liked.

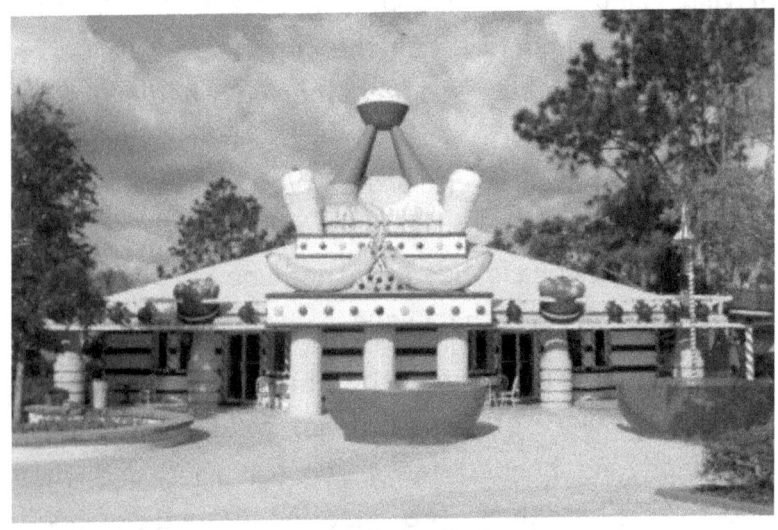

The Ice-Cream Parlour

We were full when we had finished our ice-creams but even so Michelle convinced me to go back and have another one - we just had to try the cookie-dough one!

That night Daddy and Michelle were very tired. There was so much to see and do. We were told that there would be a shuttle arriving early the next morning to take us to Disney World. Mommy was asked to go the reception area where they would have a meeting with her to explain how the village worked. Daddy went for a nap and Michelle and I played with the remote control boats. After about an hour Mommy came out of her meeting, they had explained to her what times meals would be served. We were allowed to visit one Disney park each day, but we had to make sure that the lady at reception knew which park we wanted to visit on which day.

They explained that a shuttle would arrive just after breakfast to take us to Disney World. We had to make sure that we did not keep them waiting. Each day we would find a newsletter on our dining room table, which would explain the happenings for that day in the village, as well as telling us which Disney character would be visiting the village.

They told Mommy that there was a mayor (a bunny) and his wife (a mouse) of the village who would visit us. On the last night that we were there, we would have to book a time that we wanted the mayor to kiss Michelle and I goodnight. We were given free tickets to go to Disney World. Each day I would have to wear a special pink badge that had my name on it and the **Give Kids the World** logo. This would make sure that I was given special treatment in all the parks, I would not have to stand in any queues and would be given certain free things in Disney World like photos with Disney characters. That night, before we went to sleep, we all sat on Daddy and Mommy's bed and discussed which parks we would like to see. We had no idea what was in each park, so we just randomly chose them. Michelle, Mommy and I walked to reception to hand in the form and Daddy went to sleep. Our house was so cosy, there was a huge jacuzzi in the bathroom. Before going to sleep Michelle and I decided to test drive it. That night we all slept really well because we were exhausted.

The next morning we went to the Gingerbread House for breakfast. The helpers there were very interested in us and asked us where we came from. They said we had strange accents. But Mommy was battling to understand them. There was so much food for us to choose from: bacon, eggs, sausages, tomatoes, mushrooms, onions, toast, cereals, and lots of different kinds of fruit, pancakes, waffles and crumpets. The food was delicious and we could hardly move when it was time to catch the shuttle. We had decided to go to Magic Kingdom that day.

The shuttle was waiting for us at the reception area. Some other people climbed in and we drove for about twenty minutes before we saw a huge sign saying "Disney World". I could not believe that my dream had come true.

We got off the shuttle in an enormous parking lot. From there we walked to a ferry, which carried us over a lake to the entrance of Magic Kingdom. The man at the ticket office saw my special badge and allowed us all through the gates. He asked me if I wanted to use a wheelchair. Mommy decided that would be a good idea, my leg was still a bit sore. Everybody else had to queue and pay for their tickets. I felt so special. He also gave us a map, showing us exactly where everything was.

In front of us was the beautiful Magic Castle, it was huge and towered up into the sky. As we got there, a show started. Mickey and Minnie Mouse appeared along with hundreds of dancers all dressed up in beautiful blue and white costumes. They danced and sang the happiest songs. When the show was over we started a long walk. There were shops everywhere, all selling

Disney things. We looked in a couple of shops and then decided not to waste too much time there and rather to go on the rides.

Before we knew it, it was past lunchtime. Nobody was hungry, everything was just too exciting. Mommy and Daddy took turns pushing me in my wheelchair. Magic Kingdom had many little hills so I think they got quite fit. I was too young to go on some of the rides but Daddy and Michelle went on them. Mommy came with me on others. Every now and then we met a Disney character. I had many photos taken with Cinderella, Beauty and the Beast, Sleeping Beauty and many more.

While we were sitting at a restaurant, eating the biggest hotdog we had ever seen, we suddenly heard some very loud music. A few people started to clear the streets because a parade was to start. Some of the local schools were taking part in the parade. Everybody was so excited and gathered around to watch. When they had finished we went on more rides.

Later that evening just before the park closed there was another huge parade. All the Disney characters were there, dancing down the road in front of us. There were hundreds of people watching. I wished we could stay there forever.

Never let the fun end

After the parade there was a huge fireworks display over the Magic Castle. The fireworks were in the shape of Mickey Mouse faces, stars, lips in the most beautiful colours.

We caught the shuttle back to the Village and after a delicious supper we were invited to a Pirates and Princesses Party. Daddy and Michelle were exhausted and went to sleep. But Mommy and I refused to miss out on anything. Each kid was allowed to dress up in either a Pirate or Princess costume. I was the only girl who chose a Pirate's costume. They put an eye patch on me with a bandana around my head, painted my face and then gave me a cutlass. The party was taking place in the middle of the Village. Mommy and I walked around from stall to stall. Each stall had something different. In the one I had to make my own treasure map, in another I had to find the hidden treasure. It was all so much fun. We met another family that was also from Africa, they were from Nigeria. We chatted for a long time and then walked home to our house. We were very, very tired.

The next morning we were up early and went for breakfast. After that we walked around the Village and found a mini putt-putt course, each hole had a huge dinosaur close by which either made a scary noise as you hit your ball into the hole or a whole lot of smoke would come out of his mouth. It was so exciting to play and find out what was going to happen at the end.

Then we went to Julie's Safari Theatre where we met Mickey and Minnie Mouse. They took photos of us and chatted to us.

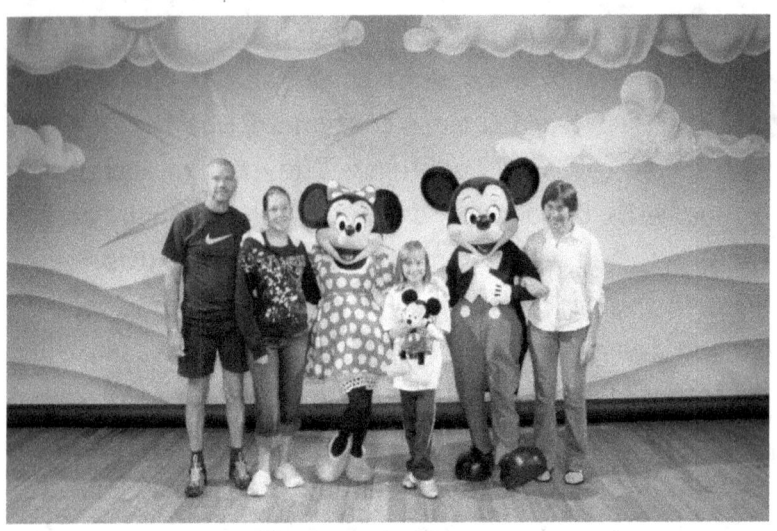

All of us with Mickey and Minnie Mouse

When we had finished we were met by Goofy outside the theatre. We could not stay long as the shuttle was waiting to take us to Animal Kingdom. Daddy and Mommy were talking in the shuttle saying that we all knew what wild animals looked like, so we would not be

Never let the fun end

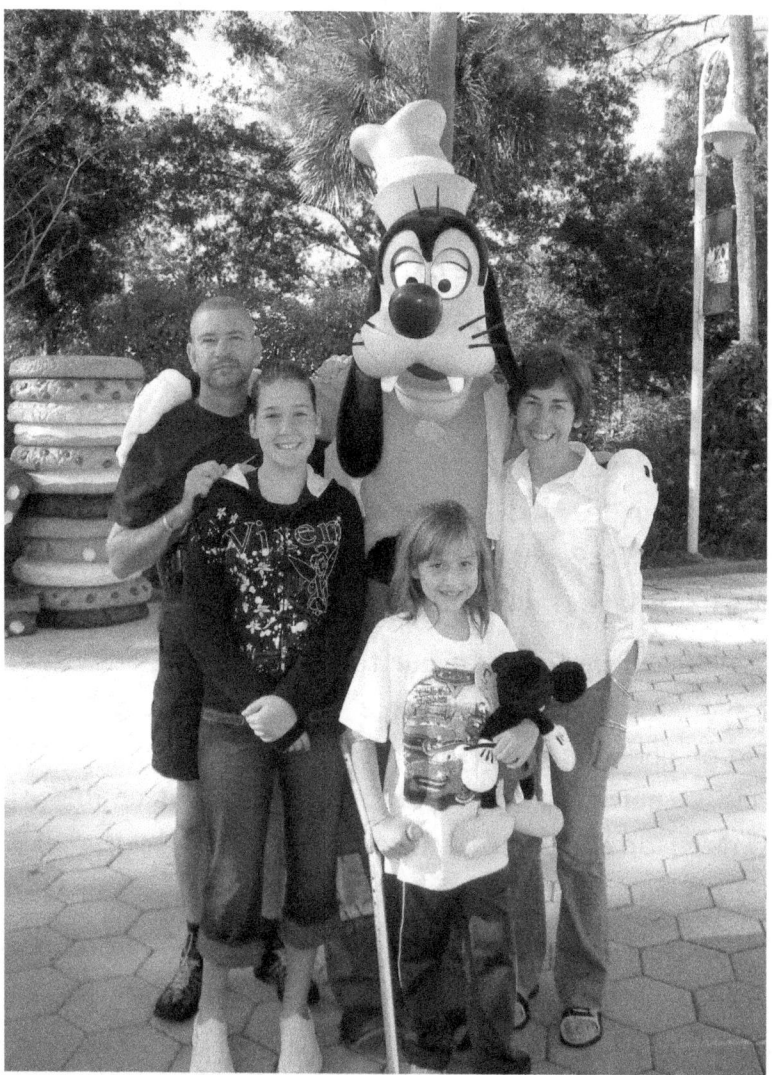

We met Goofy

staying at this park for the whole day. Maybe in the afternoon we could go to another park. We all imagined it to be a big zoo but we were in for a big surprise.

As we got through the gates, we collected my wheelchair and walked up to a huge tree in the centre of the park. Only when we got closer did we see that in the trunk of the tree were many beautifully carved animals.

Animal Kingdom was not a big zoo like we thought, although there were some animals which we had never seen before. In another section there were many exciting rides and lots of shops selling Disney stuff. Around every corner there were Disney characters waiting to meet us.

We all met our favourite characters, Daddy met Eeyore, Mommy met Winnie the Pooh, Michelle met Piglet and I met Tigger. We took lots of photos and had so much fun. Daddy and Michelle went on lots of water ride and came back soaking wet with huge smiles on their faces.

That night before the park closed, there was a huge parade. People drove multi-coloured animals made of wood, ropes and wheels in the streets of the park. There was loud party music playing. We sat on the side of the road watching for ages. There were so many people that Mommy was battling to get enough space to take photos. Soon the sun had set and it was time to go back to **Give Kids the World**.

After supper in the Gingerbread House we were invited to meet Shamu the whale, Mayor Clayton and his Wife the Mouse. There was music and many games to play. Mayor Clayton and his wife drove the cutest little yellow car. Their costumes were beautiful.

That night we visited the Ice-Cream Parlour again and after that we found Mama Merry's Pizza Kitchen just behind the Park of Dreams Pool. We could order any kind of pizza and eat as much as we liked. We were so full after that.

The next day we were going to Sea World, Mommy had really been looking forward to this park. Before we caught the shuttle we wandered through the Castle of Miracles. Outside I had a ride on the Big Carousel. Some of the people who worked at the Village were there to help me on and off the horses. They buckled up a big leather belt around my waist before the carousel started. I enjoyed it so much that I told Mommy that I had to have a ride every day before we left.

Inside the castle we saw a huge grandfather clock, a wishing well that burped, a games room and another hall full of magic. Then we found the Magic Pillow Machine. On the front of the machine we had to choose what kind of pillow we wanted by pressing different buttons, then when we pressed 'start' and a whole lot of feathers flew up and our own special pillow dropped out the machine. My pillow was a red one with Spongebob on it and Michelle's was pink with sheep on it.

On the shuttle going to SeaWorld we all felt a bit sick. Maybe it was the overeating and the fact that we were all very tired. Each day was filled with so many things to do and so much excitement. In SeaWorld, we saw many different creatures that we had never even heard of. My favourite were the manatees, they were such slow moving creatures and had the cutest looks on their faces. We fed the dolphins that came up very close to us. One of the ladies who worked there saw my **Give Kids the World** badge and gave me a small box of fish to feed the dolphins. We stayed there for ages watching them.

Then we walked around the park and went on many rides. There were lots of shows that we saw that day. The first one was a dolphin show, we all sat around a huge pool and watched them do tricks. There was another show later that day with otters, seals, and walruses. But the best show of all was that evening before the park closed, was the Shamu show.

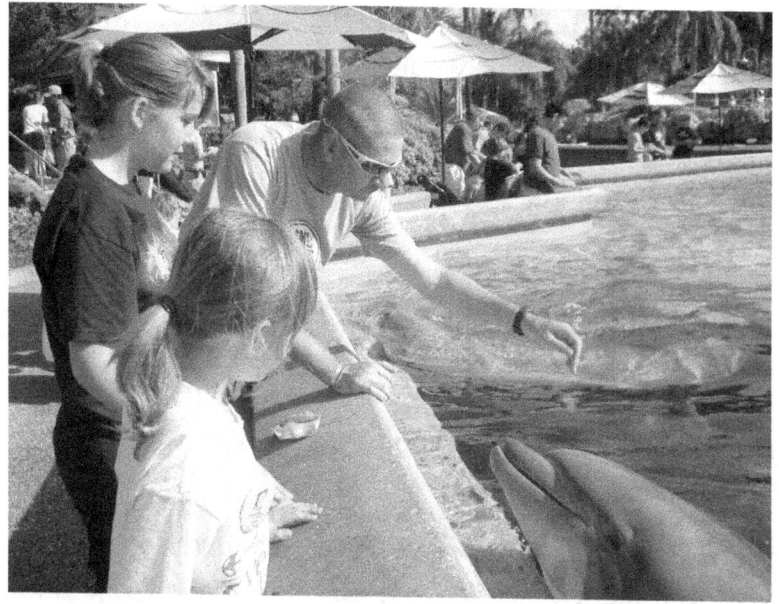
Seaworld

Shamu was a huge whale that did all kinds of tricks - it was so beautiful.

On Wednesday fifteenth November we decided to go to Epcot. I had heard that it was a sort of Science Park, I loved Science and was looking forward to it. Before we left **Give Kids the World**, I had to write my name on the little mirror star in the Castle of Miracles. First I had to give in my Star Passport at the Fairy Windows. There they scanned my personal barcode and gave me a special pen to write my name on the star. I sat at a small wooden table and wrote carefully

"Sarah 2006". Then I had to make a special wish and place my star in a magical Star Box. They told me to come back that night, the Star Fairy would be put it up along with all the other stars in the Castle Sky for everybody to see.

Before going to Epcot we all decided to pop into the Ice-Cream Parlour for a cookie dough ice cream, which was our favourite. When we got to Epcot we collected my wheelchair and a map. First we decided to visit a hall in which there were all strange kinds of Science things happening.

We did not want to waste too much time there or visit too many shops, there was not enough time in a day to do everything. Epcot was amazing. There was a water fountain but the water flowed up instead of down. Then we found my favourite ride, Test Track. Before we went on this ride, they spoke to us explaining that we were going on a ride and that our cars would be doing the same tests that are done on normal cars. We climbed into little cars, which rode around a track. As we rode we could hear a man explaining all the tests done on the cars: heat, cold, smooth surfaces, rough surfaces and we drove through them all, then we had to test the braking system. They stopped our cars and then the man counted down and our cars sped forward and suddenly stopped. After that we sped around a track at high speed and the cars rode on the sidewalls. I was a bit scared to go on this ride in the beginning but when it was finished, I begged Mommy and Daddy to go again and again and again.

There were many 3D rides, which we went on. I enjoyed the Jimmy Neutron ride, which Mommy hated. But I begged her to come on it again with me. She was really dizzy when we walked out of there.

Then Mommy found her favourite ride, E.T. Before we went on this ride we all got asked our names. Then we climbed on little bicycles and rode around trying to help E.T. find his home. At the end of the ride, E.T. thanked us all personally for helping him find his family. Mommy was the one this time who had to go on that ride three times. When we came out of this ride, they took photos of me with E.T. on his bicycle.

Around the Epcot lake, which was huge, were all kinds of different shops from all the countries around the world. Each shop had items from that country and the restaurants offered the food that was eaten there. We found a tiny little stall that had a sign outside showing 'South Africa'. We went over to see what they were selling. There was milktart, bobotie (curried mince) and curry and rice.

Spunky

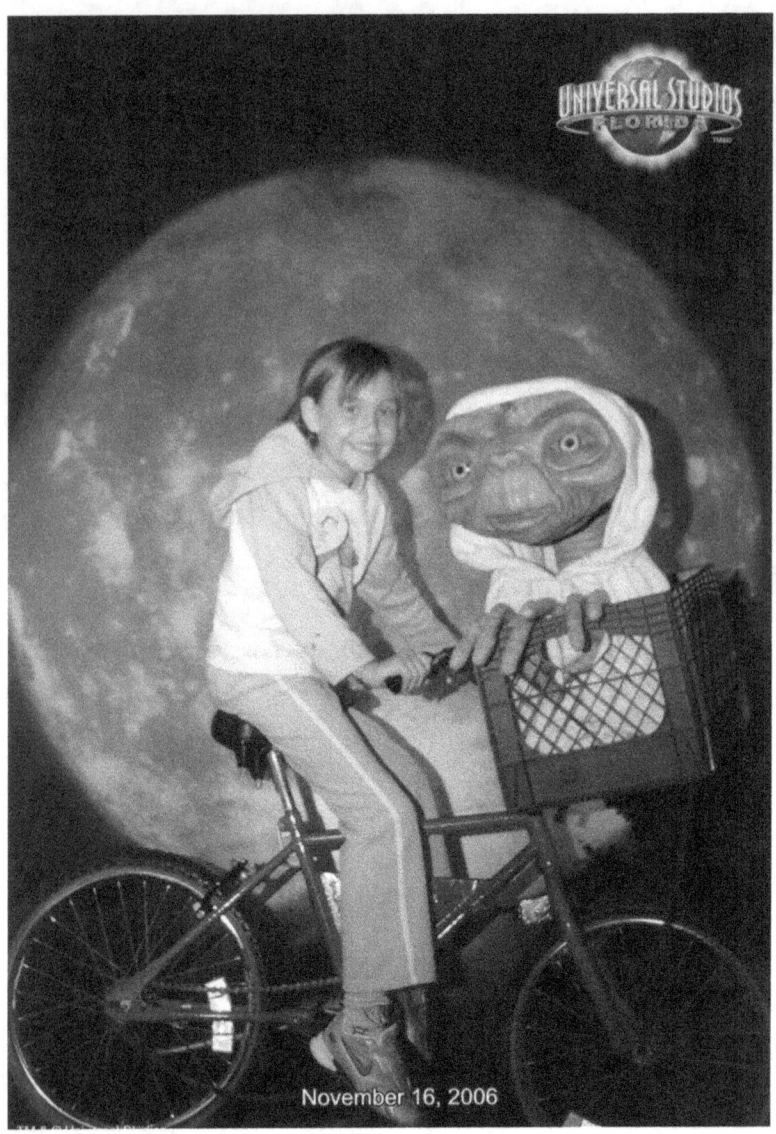

Me with ET

No biltong (dried meat) or boerewors (spicy sausage). Michelle bought some bobotie, which was delicious. We went to the man who was running the stall and told him that we came from South Africa.

We wished we could stay in America forever. Before we left Epcot we stopped at a Brazilian stall, we were all starving. Mommy and Daddy had wanted to try refried beans, which were delicious.

That evening back at the Village we went into the Castle of Miracles. A lady showed me my star on the ceiling with all the hundreds of others. A little later on, there was another party, this time it was a pie-throwing party. They dressed some people up in huge white sheets and threw pies at them, making a big mess. We played games and danced and made friends with another family. They were from Southern Carolina and their youngest daughter had leukaemia. She was still going through her treatment and looked very sick. I was so glad that my treatment was over and that I was well. They invited us to their villa for drinks. Mommy really battled to understand them because their accents were strange. They had never travelled outside their state and had no idea how far they were away from home. They were so interested to hear about South Africa and thought we lived close to Australia.

Spunky

They had three children, Michelle chatted to their eldest son and I made friends with the two younger kids. Daddy bought some biltong (dried meat) earlier in the day, it did not taste nice at all, so he gave it to the kids. They were so happy and said that their dad had never bought them such a big packet.

On Thursday we went to Universal Studios. We were told there were two different parts to this park, but we only had two more days and we still wanted to go to the MGM Studios. The parks were so big, with so much to do, we needed at least another month to do and see everything. I could not believe that our holiday was coming to an end.

My **Give Kids the World** Badge did a lot for me in Universal Studios. It was almost as if they were waiting for me. Spiderman hopped out of nowhere and asked me for a photo with him. He chatted to Mommy and I for ages while Daddy and Michelle went on a scary ride. I bought a Spiderman ball, it was a little ball connected to a piece of elastic on my wrist. I loved it and bounced it everywhere.

Then the X-Men arrived, they were very scary and did not smile at all. Wolverine had his huge steel spikes coming out of his wrists, which we wrapped around me as Mommy took a photo.

Never let the fun end

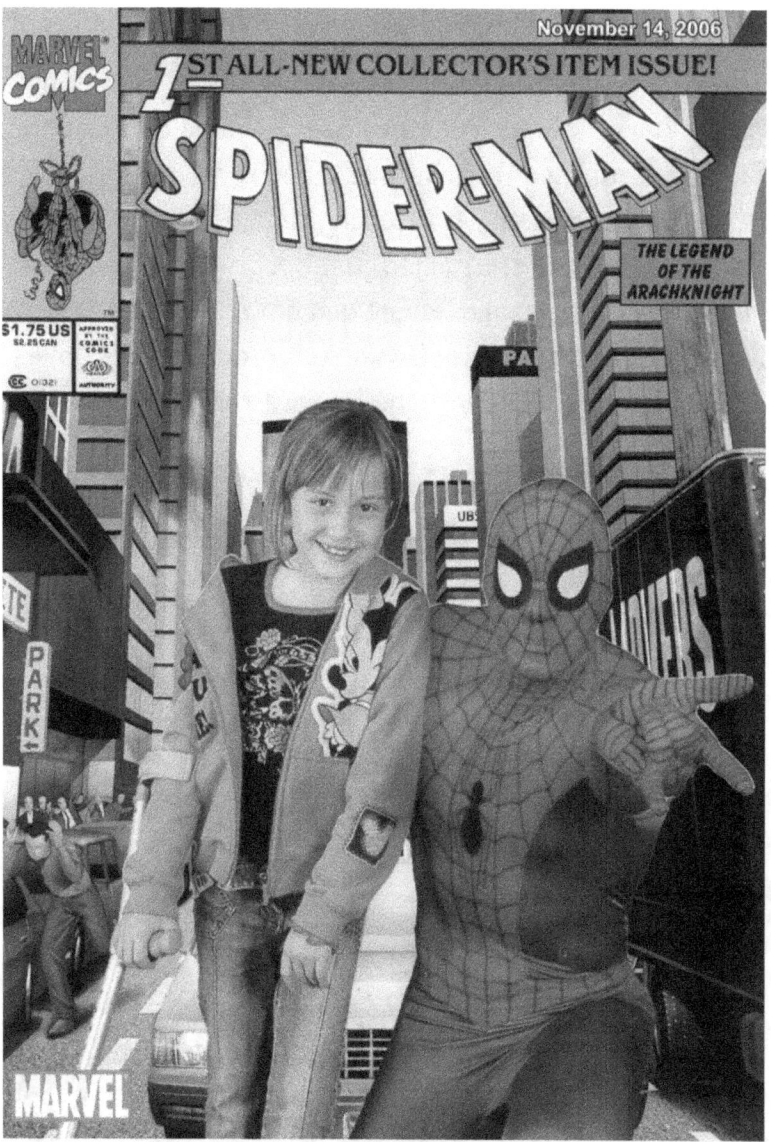

I love Spiderman

Spunky

There was so much in this park, that looked so real, but it was only a backdrop like being in a movie.

My favourite was meeting Shrek, Fiona and Donkey. Fiona was dressed in the most beautiful green velvet dress. She spoke to me for a long time. I showed her the latest Barbie doll that I had just bought. She wanted to know why I was buying Barbie and not a Fiona doll. When we posed for the photo, Donkey started to crack jokes. Afterwards he asked Michelle what her name was and

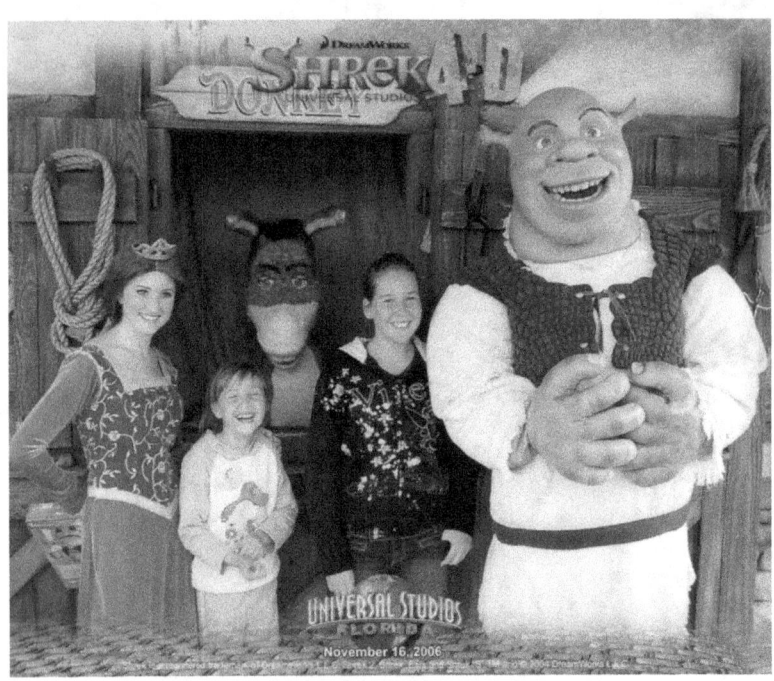

Michelle and I with Shrek, Donkey and Fiona

then asked her where she got such a strange name. We walked through the Shrek shop and Mommy bought a donkey key ring.

Daddy and Michelle had fun going on The Mummy ride and The Hulk Roller Coaster, which was a very high roller coaster.

When we got back to the Village, a Christmas party was waiting for us. Huge Christmas decorations lined the streets in the villages. A snow machine made snow and a little choir sang Christmas carols. The Mayor and his little wife were there, singing and dancing.

We had all enjoyed Universal Studios so much that we decided to go back there on our last day and see the other section of the park. Before going on the shuttle I asked Mommy if she would ride on the horse-cart with me. We had to hurry as the shuttle was leaving soon. We climbed on the cart and sat down quickly. The grey and white horses in front of us were huge, with lots of jingly bells around their necks. They started trotting slowly around the village. As we got to the reception area, we saw that the shuttle had arrived and was waiting for us. We jumped off the cart and quickly gave the horses a quick pat, thanked everybody and apologised to the shuttle driver for keeping him waiting.

We wandered in and out of the shops at Universal Studios, watched lots of shows on the sides of the streets and went on many rides. We bought many presents to take home. I found some drumsticks that lit up every time you hit them.

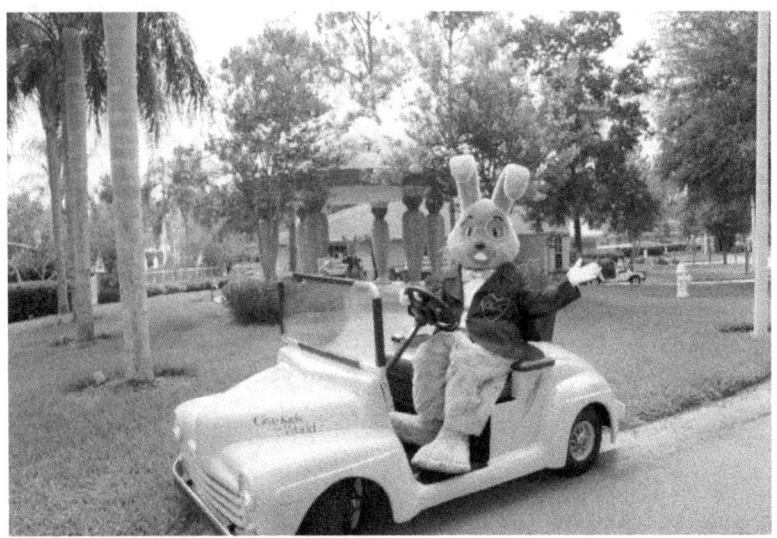

Mayor Clayton in his little yellow car

That night we had arranged that Mayor Clayton tuck us in our beds and kiss us goodnight. Mommy made sure that Michelle and I were in bed waiting for him when he knocked on the door. He was a very tall rabbit and sat on the edge of my bed.

A lady came with the mayor and asked us if we had enjoyed our stay. Mommy took photos of the Mayor kissing us goodnight. We waved goodbye as he drove off in his little yellow car. I would remember this fun village forever.

The next morning we had to get up early to catch our plane home as our flight was leaving at 5a.m. We were all sad to leave America and thanked everybody for our stay. As the plane flew over Africa, there were lots of clouds and the ride was bumpy. I felt sick but the air hostess wanted us to stay in our seats. Mommy explained to her that I needed to vomit. We spent most of that flight walking up and down to the toilets. We were all tired when we got home the next day at 3.30p.m. It was great to see our pets again but I will really miss America and all its fun.

My favourite sport

When I went for my next check up at the Joburg Gen, the doctors and nurses asked me all about our trip to Disney World. All my blood counts were fine, I had put on a little bit of weight (I now weighed 25kg) and grown slightly taller. My leg still gave trouble and whenever it was too sore, I used my crutches. My bad leg was not growing because of the damage the radiation did, so my legs were a different length. I wobbled a bit when I walked.

At school I desperately wanted to play badminton. Every Tuesday and Thursday I would watch my friends play. One afternoon I went to the teacher and asked her if I could join in. She said that she was too scared as I was still on crutches and did not want to accept responsibility if anything went wrong. I knew that I could play, I played with Michelle in the garden every afternoon and managed fine on my crutches or if my leg was too sore I would play in my wheelchair.

The next week after the practice, I asked my friend if I could knock around with her. The teacher was there and just shook her head. I was only using one crutch now, just for balance.

Spunky

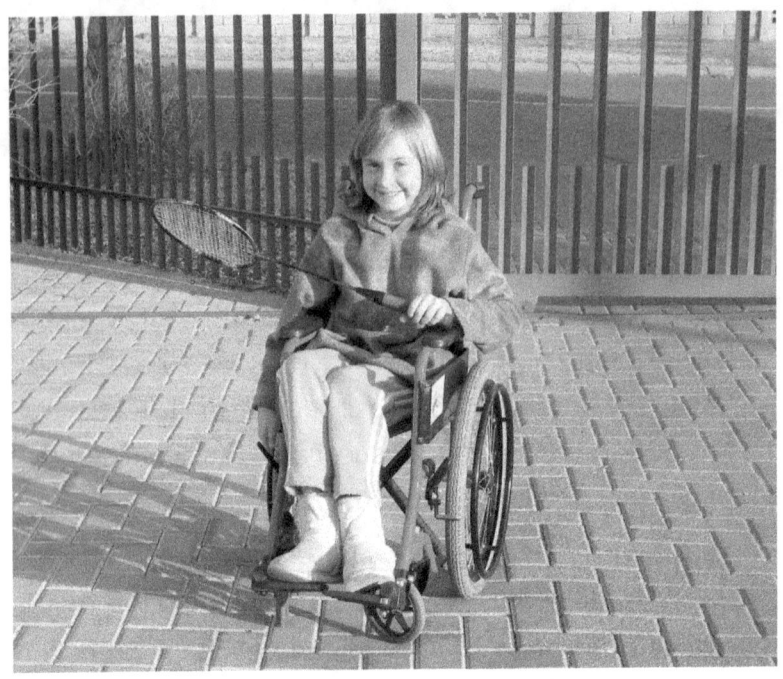

Wheelchair Badminton

The following week I nagged the teacher again, she finally agreed only if I took it easy. Mommy came to watch me and the teacher went and spoke to her. They agreed that nothing was going to stop me. I thoroughly enjoyed being part of a game and able to join in with my friends.

After a few weeks they chose the school team and I was part of it. I was not using the crutch anymore and although I could not run as fast as the others, my game was improving.

My favourite sport

At the end of that term there was an Inter-School Competition and I won all my games. Mommy came to watch me and was so proud of me.

One day Daddy went to visit one of his friends and when he came home he had a big surprise for us. His friend's dog had had puppies and he had given us one. Our puppy was brown and so cute. That night she slept in Daddy's bed. Our three other sausage dogs were not very happy with the puppy, but they soon got used to her. We decided to call her 'Jodie'. She was a cross Boerboel Ridgeback and would grow into a big dog. I made a big mistake of leaving my built-up takkies (sand shoes) out of my cupboard. Jodie was happy to chew them up. Mommy was very cross because it cost a lot of money to get my shoes built up.

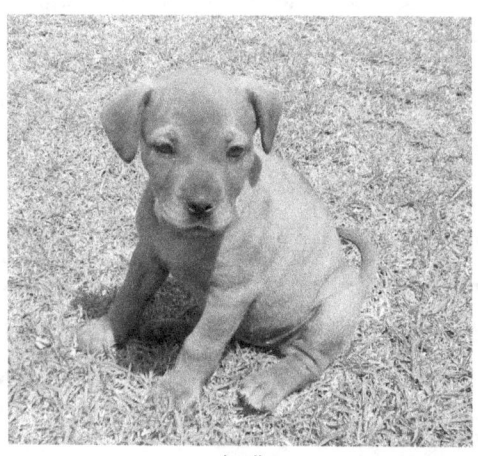

Jodie

Spunky

In the beginning of 2008 my friend convinced me to go to the Alberton Hall as there was a badminton competition taking place. We were there the whole day and I really enjoyed it. I was supposed to go back again the next day, but Mom and Dad were busy so I did not go.

The next week we got a phone call from a lady at the Badminton Club. She asked my mom why I didn't go back the next day for the rest of the competition. She explained that it was Trials to choose a badminton team to represent Southern Gauteng (a province). My mom never knew what the competition was about and apologised for not taking me back. She told my mom that I had a lot of talent and that I had played really well and that they wanted to see me play again. That afternoon when Mommy fetched me from school she told me the good news. I was so happy and could not wait for our next game.

The next meeting took place at Wanderer's Badminton Club. Mommy gave my friend and I a lift to Wanderers and watched us play. The coach came over and told her that I was playing really well. He asked her what had happened to me as he saw that I could not run properly. He was a kind man and told me that I must tell him when I got tired and that he would allow me to rest.

My favourite sport

He told us that there would be coaching at the Alberton Club every Sunday afternoon and that I must come to Wanderers every Friday evening. I was still playing at school on Tuesday and Thursday afternoons.

That Sunday afternoon they gave me the good news, I would be playing for the Southern Gauteng Under fifteen team. The six-day Tournament would be held in Bloemfontein in April. I practised really hard. Mommy worked hard at raising the money I needed for the tour.

A few weeks later my kit arrived, a very big maroon and white tracksuit, two shirts and two maroon shorts. The tracksuit was the smallest size available and I was lost in it. I was very small for my age, so we had to get it altered a lot. The tournament took place in the school holidays. I was so excited to go on tour with my friends. I enjoyed driving down to Bloemfontein with my team, we sang songs and were really looking forward to the tournament. Mommy was working from home and took a day's leave to watch me play. We had to wake up really early because the tournament started at around 8a.m. every day. We stayed at the hall the whole day and only left late at night. It was great fun but after a week I was tired and my leg was a bit sore - but nothing was going to stop me now. I made a lot of new friends and at the end of the Tournament I won a trophy for being the friendliest girl of the Tournament.

A few months later, a lady from **Moments in Time** contacted me. She wanted me to be on another calendar in 2009. They had decided to feature some people who had been in previous calendars. They used a different photo of me, which had been taken when I was going through my cancer treatment. I featured in the month of February. At the launch of the calendar in the Sandton Convention Centre, I was asked to give a speech in front of about 1500 people. It went well, although I was a bit nervous.

At the end of that year, I was entered into the Under seventeens South African and Inter-Provincial Badminton Tournament. It was held in Durban in November. Mommy came along and helped with the organisation of the tournament. I was nervous in this Tournament as the kids were a lot older and played so much better. But afterwards I realised that playing with older kids gives you a lot of experience and my game improved a lot. At the end of that Tournament, I received a trophy for Sports Girl of the Tournament and got a standing ovation.

My favourite sport

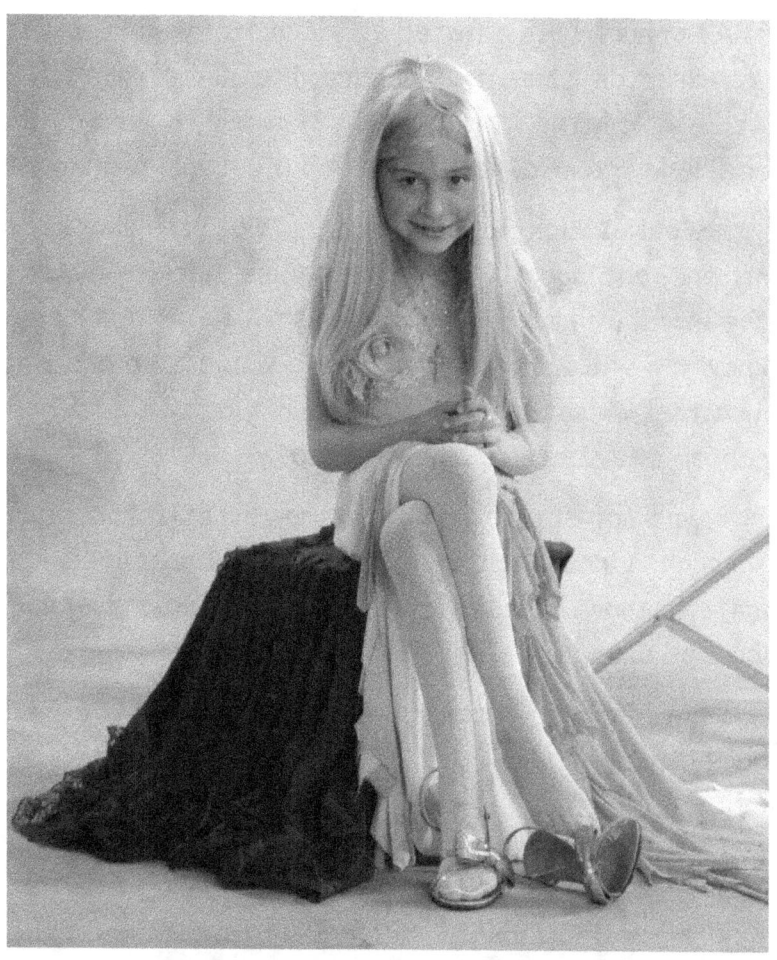

Me on the Moments in Time *calendar 2009*
Photo by Jeanne-Claire Bischoff

Spunky

At school I was invited to Honours Evening. I was called up on stage and handed the KFC Trophy for Achiever of the Year. The next week there was an article in the local newspaper about my achievements.

I started High School in 2009. I was very short for my age, and again I had some people mocking me for the way I walked. I knew that many of the kids never knew my story. Sometimes people would stop and ask me why I walked funny. As soon I explained that I had cancer, they became embarrassed.

I was not shy to let them know what I had been through. Once the teasing got quite bad and a kid imitated how I walked. The other kids joined in and laughed at me.

I put him in his place quickly by saying "Did you ever have cancer?"

He was confused and replied "No."

"Well I did, so stop mocking me." Everybody quickly stopped laughing and walked away.

At school I wrote this poem about my cancer:

A girl, a poem about me
A Girl, an ordinary girl, who believes in herself
I've been through more than you think,
I am brave!

My favourite sport

I've looked uglier than before,
But I've never seen ugly,
So I am pretty
I've never lifted a rock,
But I've lifted others spirits,
So I am brave
Don't tell me I'm not brave,
Not pretty,
Or not strong,
Because I'm a girl, an ordinary girl,
Who believes in herself
I've had cancer,
I've seen others die around me.
I've looked death in the eyes,
But I've conquered it
I've helped others who wanted to give up,
I gave them encouragement and the will to live
So we've beaten it together...
We've BECOME ONE!!!

Later that year, I was entered into the Inter-Schools Badminton Tournament in Bloemfontein. We went down in the school bus and had a huge amount of fun. My school came second in the Tournament.

In September, I entered my second South African Under fifteen Tournament, this time it was held in Pretoria. Mommy came with; she was a Manager for the B Team. I was in the A Team and doing really well. I found it quite frustrating because I wanted to be able to move faster on the court. The other kids would see me battle a bit and would make me run. They would often drop the shuttle into a part of the court that I would never be able to get to.

After a checkup at the hospital, the Oncologist advised that I see a Biokineticist to help strengthen all the muscles in my body, which would also help with my badminton. We went for daily sessions at the

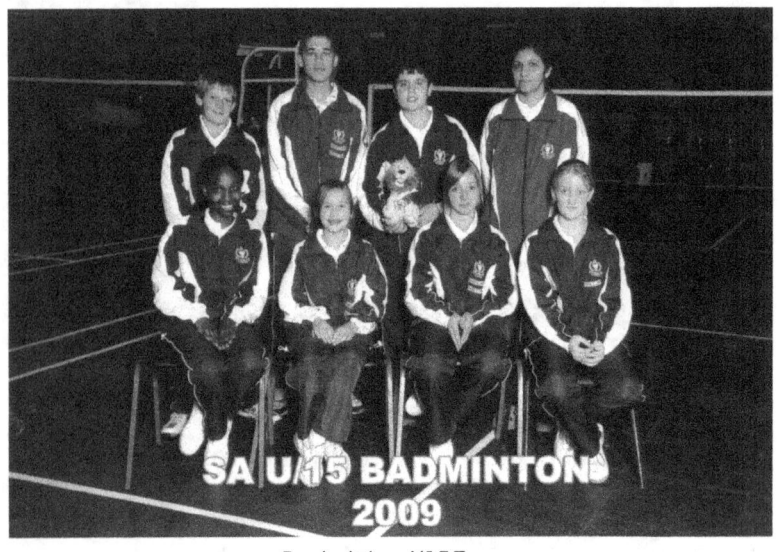

Badminton U15 Team
Bottom row second from the left

My favourite sport

Biokineticist for many months. I did many different exercises and my balance improved a lot.

In October 2009 I had my fourteenth birthday. We had a big party at home and also celebrated that I had been clear of cancer for five years. The Oncologists said that after five years my cancer would probably not return. The party went on until late at night.

After a few months my right knee started getting really sore. I fell at school and could not walk. Mommy came to fetch me. She carried me to the car and took me to casualty at the local hospital. There they put me in a wheelchair and a doctor had a look at me. He sent me for X-rays and afterwards checked my knee. He referred me to an Orthopaedic surgeon. Mommy told him that Dr Richards was my doctor, so we made an appointment and went to see him.

He looked at my knee and pressed on it. It was very sore with a lump below my kneecap. He told me that I had Osgood-Schlatter disease and would have to stop all my badminton. I could not believe what he was telling me. He explained that it was caused from overuse, especially seeing that I was playing so much badminton. He said it would resolve itself within a few weeks.

I climbed into the car in tears. I was so angry, how could he just tell me to stop playing my favourite game.

Mommy explained that it was only for a while and that I would be able to play again when my knee was better.

After a few months I was still battling with my knee. I had stopped all badminton and it was still very sore. Mommy took me to see Dr Nick who referred me to the Orthopaedic Centre. I went to see my friend there who built up my shoes. My good leg was growing and my bad leg was not, so my leg length discrepancy was now 65mm. He checked my knee and made a special brace for it. This definitely helped to support my knee, but the pain remained. He told me to use crutches again.

At the end of that year I was invited to Sports Honours Evening at school. During the awards they read out my story and I received a trophy for Extraordinary Achievement under Difficult Circumstances. I was still on crutches and could not get up on stage, so they handed me the award next to stage. Everybody stood, and with tears in their eyes gave me a standing ovation. Afterwards I was surrounded by people, congratulating me and telling me what an inspiration I was. Michelle also got two awards that night; one for Most Improved Badminton Player and one for the Captain of the A Team. Mommy and Daddy were so proud of us.

I was still going for cancer checkups which were now every six months and the Oncologist would also check out my knee. I kept on bugging them to let me play badminton again, but they told me to rest it and only go back when I am completely healed.

I was upset and just wanted to play again. I refused to even watch my friends play, it was not the same. I wanted to fly with the shuttle again.

Badminton practice began early in 2010. I desperately wanted to start again, but the teacher refused to let me. The Inter-Schools Tournament came and went, without me in it. I was so angry.

In March that year we got some bad news. My friend, Ronel from the **Moments in Time** project, who had done my make-up for the photo shoots had drowned. Her car had been swept off a bridge in pouring rain and she was unable to get out of the car in time. I was very upset as over the years we kept in regular contact. I still think about her often and miss her a lot.

Then the SA Under Nineteen Tournament started. All my friends were playing in it and I should have been there. It was a difficult tournament as the kids were much older and the games were a lot harder. I knew I would never win any of the games but I still wanted to try. I desperately wanted to play again but my knee was still too sore.

Spunky

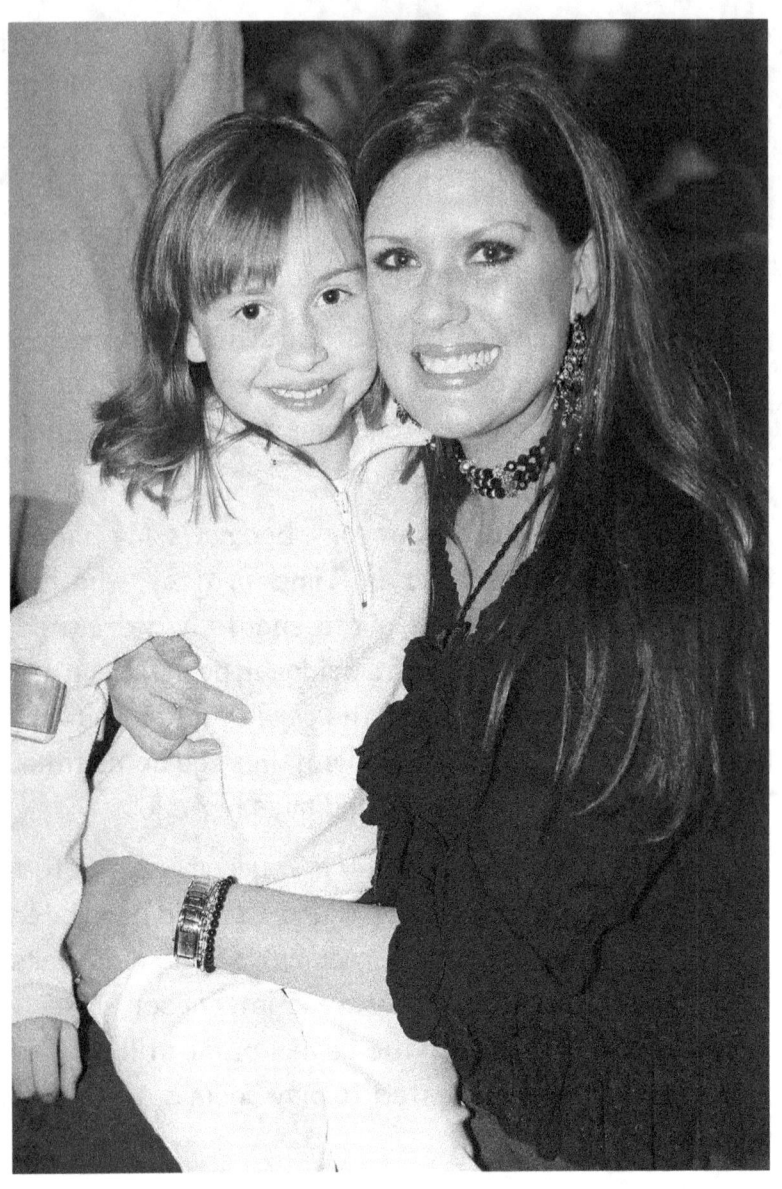

Me and Ronel

My favourite sport

In July, after much begging and pleading, I started playing at Wanderers again. Within the first few minutes of warm-up exercises, I was on my way to the Casualty Department at the hospital. I had fallen on my wrist while running backwards. In the car I was in tears, my wrist was so sore. At the hospital they took X-rays and said that I had broken my wrist. They put a wrist brace on it and told me to rest it for six weeks.

So again, I was forced to stop playing. Six weeks later, I had a check-up with another Orthopaedic surgeon who checked my wrist. He sent me for X-rays and said that it had healed very well. I could stop using the wrist brace and could go back to badminton. I was happy again.

One of my mom's customers phoned her one day and told her that she had seen a program on TV about people with different leg lengths. She had taped the program and we went to her house to watch it. On the program there was a little boy who also had legs of different lengths and he had been operated on by a doctor in Cape Town. He was perfectly even after his operation and walked normally. I really wanted to be like him. The next day Mommy phoned Doctor Peters and spent ages on the phone telling him my story. He said that I should see him.

In October 2010, I was chosen for the South African Under seventeen's that were held in Cape Town. Mommy phoned Dr Peters and made an appointment for me to see him while we were there. I was excited to see Uncle Andrew and Aunty Sharon again. While the badminton tournament was taking place, I stayed with the team and Mommy went to stay with Uncle Andrew. They came to watch me play every day.

When the tournament was over, the rest of the team flew home but Mommy and I stayed with Uncle Andrew and Aunty Sharon for a while longer. We did many fun things like visiting Butterfly World where hundreds of beautiful butterflies flew around us and landed on us when we kept still. We also went to Monkey Town, which was my favourite. We walked in a monkey cage and the monkeys hopped on us and sat on our shoulders. One monkey tried to open Mommy's camera case and take out her camera! We spent a lovely day walking up Table Mountain and spent ages looking out over the whole of Cape Town. We also visited the Castle and walked along the beach.

Just before we came home, I went to see Doctor Peters. He chatted to us for a long time and wanted to know everything that had happened to me. He was very surprised to hear that I played interprovincial badminton. Then he sent me for X-rays and a bone age scan to see if I had finished growing. When we got back to his consulting rooms he measured my leg length discrepancy and asked me to walk up and down so that he could see how I walked. He told us that both my left femur and tibia were a different length compared to the right side. My total discrepancy was 65mm. He told me that he would only operate on me to make my legs an equal length once I had finished growing. He said that I still had about another year of growth left. Although I did not want to have another operation I was looking forward to the day when I could buy shoes without having them built up. I bought mostly takkies (sand shoes) because they were the easiest to build up and didn't look so strange. I dreamt of the day that I would be able to wear a pretty pair of sandals and walk evenly without wobbling.

At the end of the year I was invited to the launch of the next **Moments in Time** calendar. I had been asked to give a speech about my cancer journey. To my surprise after my speech I was awarded with the title 'Princess of Queen of Hope'. This award was given to people who had been an inspiration to others. I went up on stage in front of hundreds of people and accepted the award.

My cancer checkups became annual check-ups, which was such good news. I was very well and my blood counts were excellent. My knee was getting much better and some days I could go without my knee brace.

But in 2011 my mom decided to keep me out of any interprovincial tournaments, because I was still having problems with my knee. I was cross because this would be the last year that I would be able to take part in that age group. I still played at school and in August I played in the South African Inter-schools Competition. It was held in Bloemfontein and although the weather was icy, it did not stop us from having a whole lot of fun.

You can do it – I did

A note from Mom (Nicky Strydom)

I secretly hoped they were wrong. I kept trying to convince myself that they would walk in and tell me that they had swapped Sarah's results with somebody else's. After all this was the Joburg Gen, the hospital that had a bad reputation. But it was the only hospital in our area with a Paediatric Oncology unit. Nevertheless, we soon were amazed at the excellent treatment we received there.

When Sarah started her first block of chemo a few days later, I was still in denial. I even wondered how I would react if they told me it was a huge mistake. I would be angry but very relieved that my child was actually fine. However, in the back of my mind I knew there was something very, very wrong, that lump on her leg that had appeared too quickly and had grown too fast.

I kept convincing myself that it would not be cancerous and soon everything would go back to normal. She would go back to riding her bike, running around and playing netball at school. It was only when Sarah's hair fell out, that reality set in. Never before, had I cried for an entire weekend. When the tears finally ended, the questions started. How could my child have cancer? She did not feel sick and definitely did not look sick. How did it start? Was it something she had eaten? Was it hereditary? What was chemo? How long was her treatment? Could she go to school? The list went on and on. Nobody I spoke to seemed to know much about Ewing's Sarcoma. So I turned to the internet, not knowing if I was reading fact or fiction. The more I read, the more I cried.

The next visit to the Joburg Gen must have been a nightmare for the Oncologists, as all my questions poured out. Patiently they answered each question over and over again as the answers weren't really making sense. Everything in my head was a huge muddle.

Over the next couple of weeks the tears stopped. I had cried myself dry for a while, but the questions never seemed to end. By this time I had read up a lot on cancer, radiation and chemo. By talking to other parents in the Oncology ward, I had discovered that a lot of them had experienced the same emotions as I had, although their children had different kinds of cancer and their treatments were different to Sarah's. We had become a small family, with tears and questions being the common ground.

Many parents left our little circle; some of their children had completed their treatment and we saw them less frequently, only when they came in for their check-ups. I envied them and hoped that one day I would be in their shoes. Other parents left our group as their children had passed away. They left a huge gap and we spoke about them often, crying together and hoping that our children would be the lucky ones. I could not bear to think of how they coped without their children, and then the tears started again. I knew that our destiny was not in our hands but hoped to sway things somehow. We were extremely lucky that we had caught Sarah's cancer in its early stages.

A note from Mom (Nicky Strydom)

That was a good thing, but we still had to be really careful that she did not pick up any infections. Many of the children who passed away, did so because of infections. So a new monster appeared, one that had to be avoided at all costs. But as part of our circle left, there were always the 'newbies', full of questions and tears. We felt like the 'old kids on the block', ready to share our experiences and ready to show the 'newbies' around.

As Sarah's treatment continued, my only wish was that Sarah would be cancer-free. I would deal with anything else that came along. I was not bothered that her leg would always be weak, that it would have severe scarring from the radiation burns or that she would vomit enormous amounts from the chemo.

At times it was very difficult for Sarah to realize her limitations, she always hoped that she would go back to 'normal'. After the removal of her tumour and the majority of muscles in her thigh, she asked me when the muscles would re-grow and when she would be able to run the way she used to, without pain or disability. Explaining that this would never happen as muscles cannot regrow, was difficult for us. She pushed herself to the limit and was soon playing badminton, much to the doctor's surprise. She would only stop when her leg or knee forced her to stop. She became irritable when this happened and would nag the Orthopaedic surgeons to let her train again. It was very difficult as I knew that her little body was taking strain but her mind was very strong.

During her treatment, I was amazed to learn how my little eight year old had touched so many people's lives. We were constantly hearing about far away people who had heard about her and how they were thinking and praying for us. We received small gifts from people that were total strangers. Even to this day, eight years later, I still get phone calls from people wanting to know how Sarah is. She became an inspiration, just as those survivors before us, had been an inspiration to us.

We, as a family, are enormously grateful to all the Doctors, Oncologists, Nurses, teachers, friends, family and strangers who helped and encouraged us throughout Sarah's treatment.

Spunky's after thoughts

I personally thank you for reading this book, and I hope as you read it, you enjoyed it. I wrote this book, not for fame, money or popularity, but to teach you all the lessons I have learnt. After reading this book, I want you to appreciate everything you have, even the smallest things.

To all the Cancer Patients out there, who are going through their treatment at the moment, or experiencing the fear that comes with it, don't give up. Each person lives in their own world. When you look out the window, you see beautiful flowers, trees, birds, but when you choose to give up, everything that is beautiful dies out, and hangs low, like your self esteem, and your hope. Each person has their own belief, their own source of hope, that they can turn to. So find your source of hope, your inspiration, and use it to go through the toughest moments, because often, the tougher it is to pass, the more you learn from it, and grow from it. The world is a pretty place when you have hope, love, inspiration and appreciation.

I hope my book has helped you to see there is a brighter side to everything, and by being yourself, you are being the most beautiful person you can ever be.

It has been eight years and even though they were not easy, they just flew by. Everyday I think about what happened and how it changed my life. Recently I have wondered, what if it did not happen? I would be able to sit on my bed and cross my legs, like I used to. I would be able to ice skate, and rollerblade. Perhaps I would be at the top of my badminton career but because of my bad leg I have definitely slowed down compared to what I *could* do. If it did not happen, I would be able to play netball, athletics and take part in all the sports that interest me.

But if it did not happen, I would not be who I am today! I would not be able to inspire and help others. I would not have the guts to stand up to bullies and tell them they are wrong. I would not *appreciate* who I am, where I am and what I *can* do. I would not wake up every morning and think "Thank you God for the sun" because when I was in hospital I did not see it much. I would not say "Thank you God for allowing me to walk to the bathroom in the middle of the night", because eight years ago I could not walk. So appreciate everything you have, even the smallest things.

I am now in Grade eleven and cannot believe that my school career is nearly over. Over the years I have heard my friends complain about school but to this day I am so grateful that I am able to be at school with my friends and teachers. I am also happy that I no longer battle with a wheelchair and crutches, and although I cannot run as fast as I wish I could, I am happy to be independent.

I have changed so much. I am sixteen and I am comfortable with myself. I act and live the way I want to, the way I think is right for me.

Thank you, God bless and I love you all

Spunky

Aunty Helen

Cancer - the Big C; the poisonous snake; daytime stalker; thief in the night; sneaking up when you're not watching; snatching the very life from you without warning. It has no bias; it does not respect age or gender, race or religion; it knows no boundaries, it knows not time, it fears no-one.

And yet... it brings with it too, a teaching – the testing of faith; the shattering of perceptions; the blasting away of pride and prejudice; forcing forgiveness; demanding unity, harmony, caring and understanding.

Our niece, Sarah was challenged with cancer when she was just eight years old. Without warning this little whirlwind of energy, this little bouncing ball of light was suddenly thrust into a world of doctors, hospitals, needles, chemotherapy, radiation, pain, fear and darkness – a world that no adult would consider entering voluntarily. And here was young Sarah just one of so many children thrust onto a path that no-one would have knowingly chosen for her.

Now you and I as adults might consider weeping and wailing and collapsing in a heap... but not Sarah. Her maturity and fighting spirit were astounding. I can't remember hearing Sarah ever saying anything other than "I'm fine thank you". Come to think of it, that was a common thread among all those sick young children. A rather humbling lesson in 'the glass is half full', don't you think?

Spunky

While not wanting to trivialize Sarah's cancer in any way – no living being should have to endure what that little mite endured – but I can't help reflecting on how darkness is always mirrored by light. While Sarah fought the fight of her life, her sometimes really dark days were brightened by some of the most amazing human beings - visits from well-known celebrities, great soccer players, musicians, invites to the theatre, and come on let's face it who wouldn't be excited about being invited back stage! Oh and what about meeting the radio presenters and chatting to them live on radio? Mind you I don't think anything in her life ever will top the excitement of visiting Disney World.

Taking part in a photo shoot, learning to play the drums, learning to walk on a leg with hardly any thigh muscles… playing badminton and studying in between are just some of the activities that kept Sarah busy after she had her last treatment. Not even a leg much shorter now than the other has got in the way of her enjoyment of life – what a remarkable young lady.

Now cancer as we said, knows no boundaries and many around the patient are thrown into their own little war of disbelief, fear, worry, anger and resentment. I salute Sarah's older sister, Michelle who simply climbed on the back of that terrifying horse and rode for her life - just thirteen at the time.

Michelle became such a trooper for her parents and Sarah, cooking, cleaning, ironing – nothing was too much for her and I know her Mom and Dad are so proud of her, as are we all.

Aunty Helen

It is said that our children are only on loan to us. It's also said that God very carefully chooses the parents of children with life challenges. No doubt Sarah's parents were at the front of that queue and I can't express enough admiration for these two souls who literally carried Sarah and others in their hands throughout her illness.

I look at Michelle just about to turn twenty-one, and Sarah now sweet sixteen enjoying life to its full, I look at the rest of the remarkable children in our family and I thank God for our blessings.

Aunty Helen

Aunty Dawne

Sarah Jayne Strydom, my niece – the calm and happy baby, the cheerful toddler, the smiling little girl and, today as a healthy and beautiful teenager, still holds all those characteristics.

We were celebrating Sarah's eighth birthday at Rietvlei Zoo Farm where she was enjoying every moment of her special day when she fell down. I saw Nicky looking where she had injured herself and cried bitterly. I went over to have a look to see how badly Sarah was hurt. All seemed to be okay and I rubbed her leg where it was obviously sore. I noticed a lump on her leg and asked Nicky if that was where she had fallen. Nicky replied that it was not and that the lump had appeared a few days before. Sarah was comforted and the birthday party continued quite happily.

Nicky took Sarah to the doctor the next day to look at the lump on her leg. Everything happened so fast after that. We were told that Sarah had cancer. Cancer! This could not be right – not almost overnight.

Les and Nicky were advised to go to the Joburg General Hospital where all paediatric oncology patients are seen. There they conducted many more tests on Sarah. Their worst fears were confirmed – Sarah did have cancer. The family stopped off at our house on the way home that evening. Les had absolutely no expression on his face – he was like a walking corpse. He answered our questions in monosyllables and just stared across the lounge. Nicky did not get out of the car, so I went to talk to her. To my questions, she gave no answers - she was speechless.

My heart went out to my brother and his wife but at that time, I felt sorrier for Michelle, Sarah's sister. She was just a little girl then, and I am sure, did not fully understand what was happening to her little sister or her parents. When you are that age, the word 'cancer' does not mean very much to you – you have heard about it but it happens to other people, not to your little sister. The seriousness and the future implications, the treatments, operations and trauma held little for Michelle. I think she felt left out, not that she was. Nicky explained it all to her but I do not think the seriousness of the situation and how sick her sister really was penetrated at that time.

Treatment was started and this was horrible. The chemo made Sarah so ill, she did not eat and got thinner and thinner. Whilst Nicky spent all her time at the hospital, sleeping, eating, living there, we as a family did our best to see to the rest of her family at home. We gave support whenever we could, but we could not take the pain away – from any of them.

We all firmly believed that Sarah would get better but sometimes it was very hard. We heard about the other children who died in the hospital and this did make us pessimistic at times. We always had to be very positive even if we were not feeling so sure of the outcome. It was hard to watch a sick child and just as hard to feel the pain her parents were feeling as we were all hurting badly – with a smile that said everything will be fine!

Michelle had to take second or even third place in the daily living experiences of the family and as sorry as I felt for Sarah, I felt just as sorry for Mich who, I think was living in a bubble at the time – not fully understanding and even at times, I think, feeling a little jealous of her sister. We tried hard to include her, to take her out, to have her sleep over, anything to make her feel special as well.

It was so hard when Sarah's hair started falling out, nothing could have prepared us for this. The whole family as well as numerous friends supported the Strydom family and tried to help them cope. Sarah got so many bandanas to wear to hide the bald head. Being the happy chappy that she is, she accepted her baldness to the extent of even being proud of it!

We all went through the agony of Sarah's radiation, the leg operations and much more. I think at the end of the day, and not counting the pain, we all suffered more than Sarah, as she just kept smiling.

Speaking for my immediate family, and I am sure the rest of the family as well, we are extremely proud of how this little girl accepted her fate, dealt with all the trauma and pain to develop into the young lady that she has become. She is an inspiration to all around her. Other sufferers can take a leaf out of her book and will also hopefully come out on top.

To her parents we say *'well done'* for believing that your daughter will overcome this. And to her sister Michelle - you coped well and should be proud of yourself. Today you surely understand all that happened at that time, and have grown up as a responsible adult. You love your sister – and she loves you.

To my brother, Les and his family, may everything that comes your way in the future never have to be that traumatic and heart wrenching again.

Aunty Dawne

Things you need to do

Here are some things you need to do if you are going through cancer treatment:

- Treat any kind of infection early.
- Eat freshly cooked meals (no takeaway's) to prevent infection. Do not eat re-heated foods.
- Wash your hands before eating your food and after going to the toilet.
- Avoid crowded areas where there might be sick people, e.g. shops, schools, churches.
- Avoid salty or spicy foods (these can burn your mouth and make ulcers.) If you have mouth ulcers from the chemo, rinse your mouth with mouthwash very often.
- Never miss your follow-up appointments.
- Don't take any medicines without checking with your doctor first.
- Find out everything you can about your kind of cancer. Make sure your information comes from a reliable source. Ask your Oncologist everything you need to know, even if you think the questions are silly.
- Finish all your treatment. If you do not, your cancer might come back.

Here are some ways you can help somebody with cancer:

- Don't stare at their bald heads! They are probably not feeling well. Rather give them sympathy and help.
- Don't tease them, rather support them and make them feel as normal as possible.
- Their families also need help and support, sometimes they just need somebody to listen to.

The Saint Siluan warning signs

Saint Siluan was a Russian monk who prayed ceaselessly for all humanity.

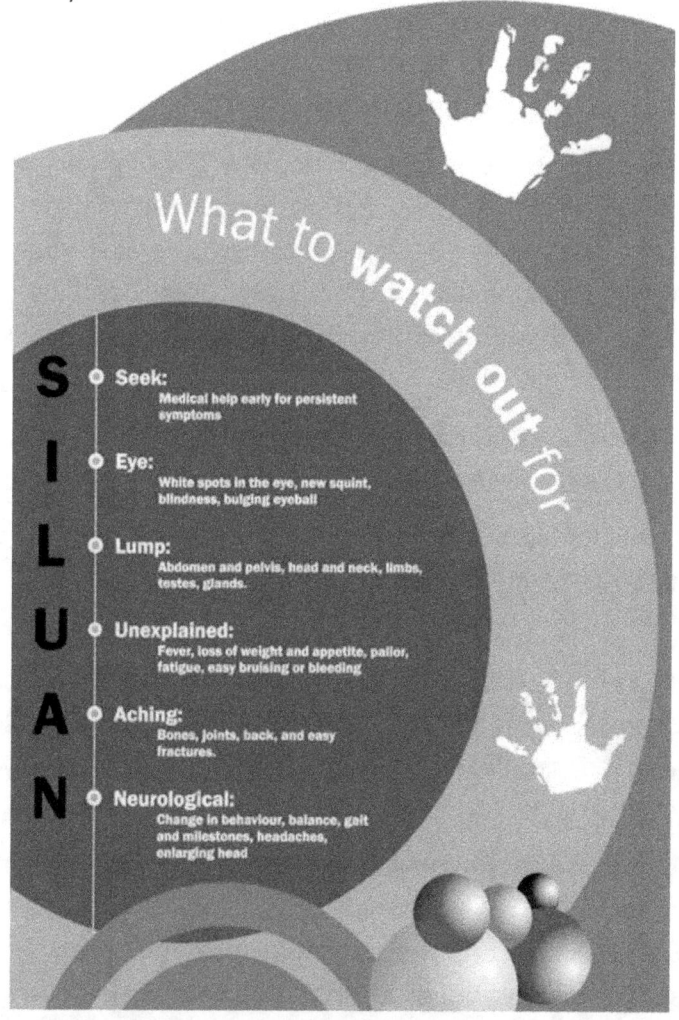

What to watch out for

S — **Seek:** Medical help early for persistent symptoms

I — **Eye:** White spots in the eye, new squint, blindness, bulging eyeball

L — **Lump:** Abdomen and pelvis, head and neck, limbs, testes, glands.

U — **Unexplained:** Fever, loss of weight and appetite, pallor, fatigue, easy bruising or bleeding

A — **Aching:** Bones, joints, back, and easy fractures.

N — **Neurological:** Change in behaviour, balance, gait and milestones, headaches, enlarging head

I would like to thank the following people from the bottom of my heart:

Our family doctor, I owe you my life. If you had not known that there was something wrong when you saw my lump and sent me for immediate treatment I might not be around today. We heard of lots of children who are misdiagnosed and they often pass away without getting the right treatment.

The fantastic team at the Oncology Department at the Joburg Gen. Thank you for giving me the best treatment to kill off the cancer. Thank you for understanding my temper tantrums, counselling me and helping me get through the toughest year of my life. Thank you for patiently answering all our questions and for all your advice.

The staff at the Radiation Department for all your help and support during my treatment.

All the doctors, surgeons, nurses and everybody who helped me through all my operations.

All the CHOC volunteers at the hospital. Thank you for the many hours you spent playing with me and all the other cancer children - for teaching us how to bead, bake, colour-in and get through their treatment in a positive way. Thank you for all your smiles that helped me so much.

All the volunteers involved in *Reach for a Dream*. A huge thank you for all the hard work you put into making my dream come true. I really enjoyed all the outings and camps. I got to do so many things that other kids can only dream about.

Give Kids the World for giving my family and me the greatest week in America with memories that will last forever.

All my teachers at school for your understanding, help, positivity and guidance, helping me to realise that I can do anything I set my mind to.

To all my family and friends, thanks so much for all the hundreds of letters of support I received, all the presents, visits and phone calls that helped me get through my treatment.

And most importantly to Daddy, Mommy and Michelle: Thank you so much for being there for me through the tough times, I know it was hard for you too but we got through it together.

Thank you for the sacrifices you had to make for me. You were all there for me and I can never thank you enough for making the right decisions, helping me, understanding me and being my best friends. I will love you forever and ever. You mean the world to me.

Notes

Some names in my book have been changed

Permission has been given to use information from: St. Siluan's Warning Signs

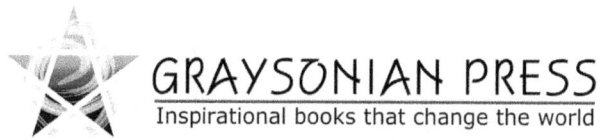

GRAYSONIAN PRESS
Inspirational books that change the world

Published by **Graysonian Press**

For a catalogue of our books:

South Africa +27 11 431 1274 (08 3610 1113)

Australia 0450 260 348

www.graysonian.com

pat@graysonian.com

Copyright © Nicky/Sarah Strydom 2012

Layout and Cover design by Ian Stokol

Outside back cover photo by Candice van der Schyff

ISBN 978-0-9872816-2-3

www.ingramcontent.com/pod-product-compliance
Lightning Source LLC
Chambersburg PA
CBHW051430290426
44109CB00016B/1495